Complete Guide to YOUTH FITNESS TESTING

Margaret J. Safrit, PhD
The American University, Washington, DC

Human Kinetics

f Congress Cataloging-in-Publication Data

Safrit, Margaret J., 1935-
    Complete guide to youth fitness testing / Margaret J. Safrit.
        p.   cm.
    Includes bibliographical references (p.) and index.
    ISBN 0-87322-757-3
    1. Physical fitness for children--Testing.   I. Title.
    GV443.S19   1995
    613.7'042--dc20   94-30281
                                                CIP

ISBN: 0-87322-757-3

Copyright © 1995 by Margaret J. Safrit

Developmental Editor: Mary E. Fowler; **Writer:** Patricia Sammann; **Assistant Editors:** Anna Curry, Erik Dafforn, and Henry Woolsey; **Copyeditor:** Anne Meyer Byler; **Proofreader:** Kathy Bennett; **Typesetter & Page Layout:** Julie Overholt; **Text Designer:** Judy Henderson; **Photo Editor:** Karen Maier; **Cover Designer:** Jack Davis; **Photographer (cover):** Will Zehr; **Photographer (interior):** Karen Maier; **Illustrator:** Tom Janowski; **Printer:** United Graphics

Printed in the United States of America   10 9 8 7 6 5 4 3 2 1

Human Kinetics
P.O. Box 5076, Champaign, IL 61825-5076
1-800-747-4457

Canada: Human Kinetics, Box 24040,
Windsor, ON N8Y 4Y9
1-800-465-7301 (in Canada only)

Europe: Human Kinetics, P.O. Box IW14,
Leeds LS16 6TR, England
(44) 532 781708

Australia: Human Kinetics, 2 Ingrid Street
Clapham 5062, South Australia
(08) 371 3755

New Zealand: Human Kinetics, P.O. Box 105-231
Auckland 1
(09) 309 2259

Contents

Preface

Fitness testing is an integral part of fitness education, but one that is not always well understood. When done well, testing can give students incentives for improving fitness and can help them understand and develop healthy lifestyles. But testing done without the proper preparation and without any connection to the physical education curriculum can discourage children from participating in physical activity. How many parents still remember their embarrassment as students when they couldn't run as fast as the rest of the class or do even one pull-up?

It isn't always easy for instructors to know which tests are best, either. Many fitness organizations now offer test batteries, each based on different definitions of fitness and different philosophies. It can take a lot of time to dig through them all to find the right one or ones for your situation.

To help physical education teachers and others involved in fitness education learn to use fitness testing wisely, we developed this text. *Guide to Youth Fitness Testing* helps you select the best tests and test batteries for your students and school and serves as a handbook on preparing children for testing, administering tests, and utilizing test results.

The guide begins with an exploration of youth fitness and testing. What is children's fitness and why should we be concerned about it? What purposes can testing serve? How does it fit into fitness education? Who is responsible for children's fitness?

In the next four chapters we focus on test selection. In chapter 2 we lay out guidelines for choosing a test battery, based on three main criteria: your philosophy of fitness education; the practical aspects of the battery's use; and the validity, reliability, and objectivity of the tests and test battery. Chapter 3 takes some of the guesswork out of test battery selection by giving you all the pertinent details on six of the nation's most widely used test batteries:

- American Alliance for Health, Physical Education, Recreation and Dance (AAHPERD) Physical Best Fitness Program
- Chrysler Fund/Amateur Athletic Union (AAU) Physical Fitness Program
- Prudential FITNESSGRAM
- President's Challenge Physical Fitness Program
- YMCA Youth Fitness Test
- National Youth Physical Fitness Program

Information on each includes

- the test sponsor and developer,
- the target population,
- the battery's definition of fitness,
- the tests,
- the standards and award systems,

- the materials, and
- the software.

Chapter 4 goes into further detail about each of 22 tests included in the test batteries, with information about its

- objective,
- advantages and disadvantages,
- measurement capabilities (when that information is available),
- protocol, and
- scoring.

Finally, chapter 5 helps you develop your own test battery by enabling you to choose from existing test batteries or create your own tests. The advantages and disadvantages of doing this are discussed.

The next two chapters, written by Cynthia L. Pemberton, PhD, look at test usage and results. Chapter 6 presents ideas on preparing yourself and your students for testing (including a section on children with special needs), and then explains how to administer tests more easily and with better accuracy. Suggestions for recording and analyzing results follow. Chapter 7 discusses how to best use test results. It has tips on giving feedback to children and their parents and setting goals with children. It also covers the controversial area of awards: Are they helpful? If used, which award system is most motivating? The chapter concludes with some thoughts on the use of test results in program and student evaluation.

The last chapter returns to the idea of testing as part of fitness education. It includes an annotated bibliography of resources for testing and fitness education. The appendixes offer resources for purchasing or building test equipment and provide test norms for the National Children and Youth Fitness Study (NCYFS), and criterion-referenced standards for the AAHPERD Physical Best Fitness Program, and the Prudential FITNESSGRAM program.

We hope that after you read this book you'll have a clearer idea of which tests are best for you and what they can do in your program. We also hope that you'll know how to get the most out of testing by preparing your students to do well and by using the results to promote children's fitness and to involve children's parents. Testing doesn't have to be torture, for students or teachers. Instead, it can be a vital part of your fitness curriculum.

CHAPTER 1

Youth Fitness and Fitness Testing: How Do They Relate?

Think about a playground full of children. Some are on swings, pumping their legs to reach ever-higher heights. Others are clambering on a jungle gym or pretending to be soldiers or cops and robbers. Still others are in a circle, pitching a gym ball around. It's a picture of continuous motion, and it would lead you to assume that children are naturally physically fit.

But is that true? Today some researchers challenge the notion that most children are fit. Many people believe children now watch TV too much and play less actively than children of earlier eras. Whether that's true is yet to be determined, but we do know that children's fitness is important.

In 1992 the American Heart Association Scientific Council released a position statement on exercise, recognizing physical inactivity for the first time as a risk factor for coronary artery disease, one of the main killers of Americans today (American Heart Association, 1992). Although this statement was based on research done on adults, it also has implications for children.

Physical activity is a learned behavior. For children to develop a lifelong habit of exercise, we must educate them from an early age about the importance of physical activity in maintaining good health. They must learn not only skills and fitness activities but also the principles of regular physical activity. As the American Heart Association (1992) states, "Persons of all ages should include physical activity in a comprehensive program of health promotion and disease prevention, and should increase their habitual physical activity to a level appropriate to their capacities, needs, and interest" (p. 2727).

To teach physical fitness, however, we first need to know what it is.

What Is Physical Fitness?

Physical fitness has been defined in many ways. One of the broadest definitions has been the ability to handle the tasks performed in everyday life with enough energy in reserve to enjoy leisure pursuits and deal with emergencies. Given that Americans today, at work and at leisure, are often sedentary, we believe that a more appropriate definition for fitness is the capacity of the heart, blood vessels, lungs, and muscles to function at optimum efficiency (Pate, 1983). Fitness is a physical state of well-being that allows people to perform daily activities with vigor, reduce their risks of health problems related to lack of exercise, and establish a base of fitness for participation in a variety of physical activities (Ratliffe & Ratliffe, 1994).

This latter, health-related definition of fitness is usually measured by components related to risk factors for disease. These components are often identified as muscular strength and endurance, flexibility, aerobic capacity, and body composition, although developers of major fitness tests define them a little differently.

Children's fitness has the same goals as adult fitness, but it applies to the needs of children and youth, according to their level of maturation. It is specifically developed for children, rather than an adaptation of an adult model.

Knowing *what* fitness is, though, leads to another question: Why should we worry about children's fitness?

Why Be Concerned About Children's Physical Fitness?

First, many people believe that children's fitness is tied to their later health as adults (Rowland, 1990). Evidence of elevated cholesterol levels and early stages of hardening of the arteries has been found in some children, both conditions possibly leading to heart disease in adulthood.

Physicians, teachers, and health promotion specialists also have expressed concern about children's weight. Some children become overweight at an early age. Of these, a portion may attempt to handle their weight problems through excessive dieting or purging. Others who ignore the problem may develop long-term problems with weight control, which in adulthood can expose them to such health risks as diabetes, heart disease, and stroke.

But are children at risk today because of low fitness levels? It depends on whom you talk to.

What Is the Fitness of Youth Today?

Many reports have been published about the poor fitness of youth in America, but that status remains a controversial issue.

On the negative side, several large surveillances of youth fitness, comparing the results of mass fitness testing over a decade, seem to show that American children are unfit. The National School Population Fitness Survey, published in 1985, compared its results with those from 1975 and found little change (Reiff et al., 1985). The levels in both years were low in important fitness components. Cardiorespiratory endurance and upper-body strength were poor for both boys and girls, and boys' flexibility was inadequate. Girls' scores stayed stable or declined after age 14 on most components of fitness. The National Children and Youth Fitness Studies also reported low levels of fitness in their large-scale study.

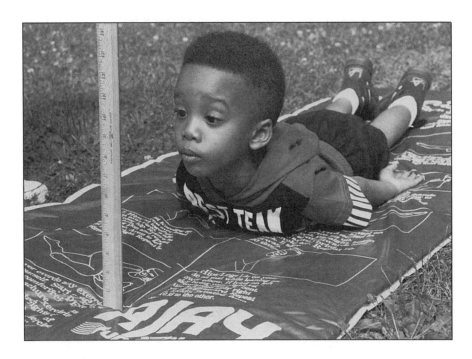

More recently, however, several proponents of youth fitness have suggested that American children are, in fact, generally fit (Blair, 1992; Blair, Clark, Cureton, & Powell, 1989; Rowland, 1990). These researchers have not questioned the results obtained in the nationwide surveys mentioned before; rather, they interpret the results differently.

Blair (1992) believes that children are generally fit. Large-scale studies of adults (Blair et al., 1989) have shown that the 20% of the adult population that is the least fit has the greatest percentage of deaths in follow-up studies. Even those in the next highest 20% of fitness have a greatly reduced risk of disease factors. Assuming that the adult data apply to children, Blair suggests it is reasonable to expect that about 20% of the children and youth in this country are unfit.

In part, researchers base their conclusions that American children are reasonably fit on the health-related standards promoted by several developers of national fitness tests (such standards will be discussed later). But we do not know whether the majority of American children are fit or unfit because those standards have not been proven completely accurate. Whatever the fitness of American children as a whole, however, is there a need for you to know the fitness of the children you work with?

Why Should I Fitness Test?

Though youth physical fitness testing may be only a small part of a larger fitness education program, it is an important one. Testing can help you

- *Track children's progress:* You can't know what you've accomplished if you have no idea where you started. You need a baseline and a measuring stick to decide where each child is and how much he or she improves over time. Fitness testing, if done properly, can perform these functions.

- *Decide on program content:* Without testing how do you know the children's strengths and weaknesses? Test results give you a place to start in designing programs.

- *Place children:* To learn, children need experiences that are not so far beyond their capabilities that they cannot succeed, yet not so far below what they can do that they are not challenged. Fitness education activities should stretch children's abilities both mentally and physically. To plan such activities, you must know what students are presently capable of doing.

- *Motivate children:* When you test as part of a complete fitness education program and children understand the components of fitness and the reasons for testing, test results can provide incentives for them to improve or maintain their fitness.

- *Promote physical education:* Test results, if presented clearly, can grab the attention of school administrators and parents. Although you must be careful to keep others from misinterpreting results or expecting more improvement over a limited time than is realistically possible, test scores offer a concrete measure of your physical education program that helps legitimize its importance.

- *Evaluate your program:* You can use test scores as one measure of your program's quality, but do so cautiously. Many factors beyond your control, such as heredity or the amount of time children are in class, can affect whether or not test scores improve.

Obviously, testing can serve many purposes, But how does it fit with the rest of a fitness education program?

What Is the Role of Fitness Testing in Fitness Education?

Actually, fitness testing can fulfill its potential only when it is based in fitness education. Test results can be meaningful to children only when they understand the basic concepts of physical fitness and how those concepts affect their lives. First graders can understand that the heart beats faster as activity level increases; third graders can understand the analogy of the heart as a pump.

Conversely, having that knowledge makes children more willing to try harder when they are being tested and to use the results to improve their fitness behaviors. And it provides the groundwork for good fitness behaviors in adulthood.

One part of fitness education is preparation for testing. A good fitness education program should not only give children the cognitive background for understanding test results but should also ensure that children know how to perform the test items and how the testing will be organized.

The testing then gives you feedback on students so you know what they need and can measure their progress throughout the year. From this knowledge should come the specific fitness activities that become part of your fitness education program.

Testing, then, is part of a cycle that moves from fitness education through test preparation and testing to using the feedback for activity planning (see

Figure 1.1). You can judge the success of those activities to some degree by later testing.

This gives us a good model for fitness education. But a final question is: Who is responsible for this education?

Who Is Responsible for Youth Fitness?

Although physical educators play an important role in teaching children about physical fitness, they can't be the only ones responsible for fitness. At the elementary school level, children may be in physical education class for only one or two 30-min periods each week. In secondary schools, junior and senior students may not even be enrolled in physical education. Thus, other community members must teach and reinforce physical fitness as well.

Parents can support appropriate exercise and nutrition, both by example and by providing encouragement and arranging to make better fitness habits possible. If parents emphasize fitness at home, the entire family can participate and benefit.

Classroom teachers, particularly at the elementary school level, can reinforce fitness concepts and activities while teaching in their content areas. In math, children could calculate running times or convert distance run scores to aerobic capacity measurements. In English, children could write essays related to exercise or other fitness topics. The entire school might participate in a fitness week or month in which all teachers incorporated fitness into their curricula.

Community youth groups also can contribute to children's fitness—church groups, Boy and Girl Scouts, the YMCA and YWCA, recreation groups, and many more. Although fitness is not a major focus in some of these groups, it could still be a part of special programs and activities.

Summary

- Physical fitness is the capacity of the heart, blood vessels, lungs, and muscles to function at optimum efficiency. It is a physical state of well-being that

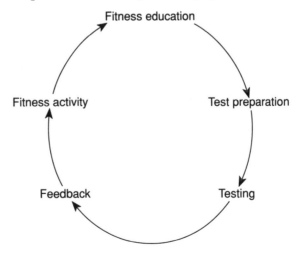

Figure 1.1   The fitness education cycle.

allows people to perform daily activities, reduce their risk of health problems, and participate in physical activities.

- Health-related physical fitness is measured by five components: aerobic capacity, body composition, muscular strength, muscular endurance, and flexibility.
- Children's fitness is specific to the needs of children and youth according to their levels of maturation, *not* just an adaptation of an adult model of fitness.
- Children's physical fitness is important because it may be tied to health in adulthood and because some children are becoming overweight at an early age.
- Whether American children are, in general, fit is controversial.
- Fitness testing helps you
  - track children's progress,
  - decide on program content,
  - place children within the program,
  - motivate children, and
  - promote physical education.
- Testing is a part of a cycle that moves from fitness education through test preparation and testing to using feedback for activity planning, which is measured by later testing.
- The community, as well as the physical education teacher, must be involved in teaching children about physical fitness. Parents, classroom teachers, and youth groups can all contribute.

References

American Heart Association. (1992). *Statement on exercise: Benefits and recommendations for physical activity programs for all Americans.* Dallas: Office of Scientific Affairs, American Heart Association.

Blair, S.N. (1992). Are American children and youth fit? The need for better data. *Research Quarterly for Exercise and Sport, 63*, 120-123.

Blair, S.N., Clark, D.G., Cureton, K.J., & Powell, K.E. (1989). Exercise and fitness in childhood: Implications for a lifetime of health. In C.V. Gisolfi and D.V. Lamb (Eds.), *Perspectives in exercise science and sports medicine: Youth, exercise, and sport* (pp. 401-430). Indianapolis: Benchmark Press.

Blair, S.N., Kohl III, H.W., Paffenbarger, Jr., R.S., Clark, D.G., Cooper, K.H., & Gibbons, L.W. (1989). Physical fitness and all-cause mortality: A prospective study of healthy men and women. *Journal of the American Medical Association, 264*, 2395-2401.

Pate, R.R. (1983). A new definition of youth fitness. *Physician and Sportsmedicine, 11*(4), 77-86.

Ratliffe, T., & Ratliffe, L.M. (1994). *Teaching children fitness: Becoming a master teacher.* Champaign, IL: Human Kinetics.

Reiff, G.G., Dixon, W.R., Jacobs, D., Ye, G.X., Spain, C.G., & Hunsicker, P.A. (1985). *National school population fitness survey* (Research Project 282-84-0086). Washington, DC: President's Council on Physical Fitness and Sports.

Rowland, T.W. (1990). *Exercise and children's health.* Champaign, IL: Human Kinetics.

CHAPTER 2

Criteria for Choosing a Testing Program

Wouldn't life be easier if there was only one national fitness test battery? Deciding among all the commercial, state, and agency fitness testing packages now available can be confusing. Also, with only one test battery, efforts to revise and improve testing could focus on that single battery.

But having multiple batteries available has some advantages, too. With these choices, you can select the one that fits your program's philosophy of fitness education and testing. We also hope that the competition among test developers will eventually lead to better tests.

If you are going to be involved in choosing a test battery, whether you're part of a committee making recommendations or are free to choose for your own program, you'll find it difficult and time-consuming to gather the necessary information on the different test packages to make an educated decision. We wrote this book to help simplify the process for you.

To choose wisely, though, you will still have to be aware of what you're looking for in a test. In this chapter we point out some of the most important aspects of test batteries to help guide you in your decision making. No test battery will be perfect, but if you are clear on what you want, you should be able to find the one that's closest to your ideal.

The first aspect of test battery selection we want to highlight is your philosophy of fitness education. Thinking about that will help you narrow the number of tests you consider. Next are the practical aspects of testing: appropriateness for your students, ease of administration, availability and quality of support materials and customer service, and cost. Finally, it's good to take into account how well the battery and the individual tests actually measure what they are supposed to measure. Are the tests, separately and together, valid, reliable, and objective? Let's consider all three of these areas.

Philosophy of Fitness Education

Your program's focus should determine the types of tests and the standards for those tests that you use. This applies not only to the specifics of the particular aspect of fitness being tested but also to the broader question of whether you want to assess children by comparing them to each other or to a set of standards.

Norm-Referenced Versus Criterion-Referenced Standards

A *standard*, in the context of fitness testing, is a number representing a desirable level of achievement on a test. Two common types for fitness testing are norm-referenced and criterion-referenced standards.

Norm-Referenced Standards

Norms represent how a group of students actually performed on a test, usually a reference group such as a nationwide sample of students. The scores of any student can then be compared with these norms.

In the past, the developers of most widely used physical fitness tests encouraged users to interpret scores based on a table of norms. Those norms were usually presented as percentiles. A *percentile* indicates the percentage of people in the reference group falling below a given score. For example, if you scored at the 85th percentile, then 85 percent of those taking the test scored below you and 15 percent scored above you.

The once popular Youth Fitness Test (American Alliance for Health, Physical Education and Recreation [AAHPER], 1976) included two tables of percentile norms, one for boys and one for girls, although no particular percentile standard was set. Students were encouraged to plot a profile chart using percentile scores each time the test was given. The test manual stated that "the 50th percentile shows the average" (AAHPER, 1976, p. 64).

The President's Challenge Physical Fitness Program (President's Challenge, 1989) has two performance standards, both based on a table of norm percentiles. The first standard is the 85th percentile, representing outstanding performance; the second is the 50th percentile, showing average performance.

Norms have a few properties that you need to know. First, norms are dependent on the set of scores used to establish them. This means that if you want to compare your students' scores with American students in general, the reference group (also known as the sample) should be representative of the national population of school-age children. Two test developers who have used scientifically chosen national samples are the President's Council on Physical Fitness and Sports (PCPFS) (Reiff et al., 1985) and the National Children and Youth Fitness Study (NCYFS) I and II group (Ross & Gilbert, 1985; Ross & Pate, 1987). If you would prefer to compare the performance of your students with other students in your town or state, you would have to test a large, scientifically selected sample of students to develop your own table of norms. (The measurement specialist in your school system can assist you with this.)

Second, tables of norms published for fitness tests are generally meant to be used to interpret individual scores, not the average score for a class or an age group. The tables themselves are based on individual scores, and the distribution of scores for individuals typically is wider than the distribution for group averages. Norms based on individual scores would underestimate group averages higher than the middle of the distribution and overestimate those lower than the middle.

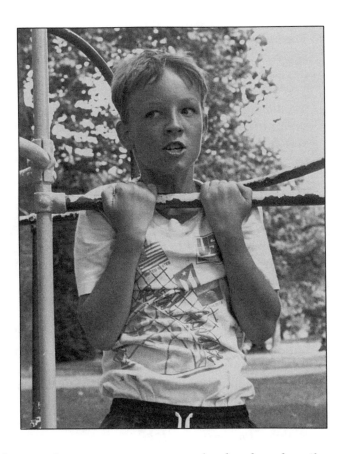

A table of norms for group averages can be developed easily, as long as the groups used to develop the table have been carefully selected. If you don't wish to do this, you can still use the information from a table of individual norms to interpret group data if you calculate the *percentage* of students in your class who exceed a specific percentile rather than comparing the group average. See an article by Spray (1977) or the textbook by Safrit (1990; pp. 425-427) for more on this procedure, as well as others.

Finally, using a specific percentile as the standard of performance may create unrealistic expectations for many students. The ability to perform at a high level on fitness tests is, in part, a function of the person's genetic makeup, so it's impossible for some students to achieve at the levels represented by the higher percentiles. This doesn't mean that norms shouldn't be used. They can perhaps be more useful, though, in program evaluation than as standards for individual achievement. For that, criterion-referenced standards are thought to be more useful.

Criterion-Referenced Standards

If you've been following the latest in physical fitness testing, you are aware that many test batteries now include criterion-referenced standards, also known as health-referenced or health standards. A *criterion-referenced standard* is based not on norms but rather on research done to set a minimal level of fitness that indicates a child is in good health.

To have a criterion-referenced standard, a test must measure some aspect of health; there must be some criterion to which performance of the test activity is related. For instance, the one-mile walk/run test measures aerobic capacity. The standard for it should represent the criterion that is the minimum level of aerobic capacity needed to reduce the risk of heart disease, which needs to be developed through research.

We need to note certain characteristics of criterion-referenced standards as we did with norm-referenced standards. First, the accuracy of the standards set for fitness tests thus far is questionable. The most valid standards probably are those for the one-mile run, and even those have some problems. Other tests, such as sit-ups and sit-and-reach, have little justification for their criterion-referenced standards. However, work is being done to improve the accuracy of standards, and the standard-setting process should improve in the future.

Second, because very fit students may meet the standards easily, they may not be motivated to attain or maintain higher levels of fitness. To counteract this, promote not only the published criterion-referenced standard but also an additional, higher standard (one you set for your class or school) for the fitter student. Reward higher levels of achievement as well as the normal standard. You can also ask highly fit students to compete against themselves, to try to better their own scores.

Finally, because criterion-referenced standards are not a function of the distribution of scores, you must determine validity and reliability for these standards. In other words, do students who meet or exceed the standard also possess the positive state of health associated with the component of fitness being measured? The test developer should provide this information in the test manual.

Which Standards to Use?

In a recent study (Koebel, Swank, & Swinburne, 1992), children's average test scores were converted to norm-referenced (President's Challenge) and criterion-referenced (Physical Best) standards and compared. On the average, no age group of either sex passed the norm-referenced standards. Only a few of the average test scores failed to meet the criterion-referenced standards. It's more reasonable to expect children to score at the 50th percentile on norm-referenced tests and at criterion-referenced standards reflecting the performance level of children at the 20th percentile. (The 20th percentile represents the point in the adult population separating high-risk and low-risk individuals.)

Generally, criterion-referenced standards are best as the *primary* standard for an individual. The emphasis in fitness testing should be to perform well enough to meet minimum health-related standards. Norm-referenced standards, however, are useful for comparing your students with others across the country or locally and for identifying high levels of achievement by individuals.

Health-Related Versus Performance-Related Tests

Test batteries can emphasize one of two types of measurements: those that are health-related, chosen to measure a component of health; and those that are performance-related, chosen to measure a motor task.

An example of a health-related test would be a distance run. The student's performance can be related to personal health because there is a direct tie

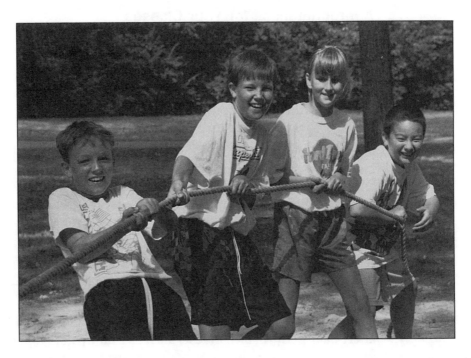

between the test score and maximal oxygen uptake, an indicator of aerobic capacity. Participation in vigorous physical activity leads to improvement in aerobic capacity and helps prevent heart disease.

A performance-related test would be a measure of grip strength. Such strength is needed for particular motor tasks, but it's not directly related to an individual's good health.

In truth, it's not possible to view a test as purely one type or the other. There's an element of both in any test of motor performance. But it can be a useful distinction. For instance, performance-related tests are helpful in sports. Consider a physical fitness test for football players. The test might include a 40-yd dash and a bench press test, but these might or might not directly relate to the health of the players. On the other hand, health-related fitness tests are appropriate for all students.

The type of standard used is affected by whether the test is health-related or performance-related. Standards for a health-related test should show what level people must achieve for minimum good health, not what a given population actually reaches, so they are criterion-referenced. Performance-related test standards can be norms that are used to identify high-level performers and are particularly helpful in sports.

Practical Considerations

Depending on what you want to measure and accomplish in your physical education program, you can choose between criterion- and norm-referenced and between performance- and health-related test batteries. After that broad separation, you still probably have quite a few test packages to choose from. The next area to examine is practical considerations. Is this battery suitable for my students? Is it easy to administer at our facility? What support materials and services are offered? And, maybe most important, what will it cost?

Appropriateness for Your Classes

You know your students' needs better than anyone else. Think about some of the following characteristics when choosing a test battery for them.

Age: Some tests, such as a one-mile walk/run, are not as motivating for young children as they are for older children. An alternative, such as the 20-m shuttle run, may be more appropriate.

Gender: Boys and girls may need different program emphases. For example, boys may need more work on flexibility, whereas girls may need to stress arm and shoulder girdle strength. Also, because of physiological differences between the sexes, different performance standards should be provided for each group.

Skill levels: For some tests, a student's level of skill may influence the results. For instance, for the one-mile walk/run, students who know how to run correctly may outperform those who don't, although their aerobic capacity may be the same. Skill might also affect tests such as the shuttle run or standing broad jump.

Individual differences: Children's differences in body weight or height might affect their performance in tests such as pull-ups or sit-and-reach. The amount of motivation each child has may also determine how much of an effort she or he puts forth.

Culture: No physiological differences are involved between cultures, but there may be social values that cause children from various groups to view fitness and exercise differently. For example, some cultures may have reservations about girls engaging in vigorous physical activity.

Disabilities: Tests often need to be adjusted to accommodate children with disabilities. Some test batteries include suggestions for altering test protocols for those with certain disabilities. (See p. 82 for more on testing children with disabilities.)

Ease of Administration

How tough or easy is it to administer the test batteries you are considering? Part of that depends on your situation, part on the tests themselves. Use these questions to guide your thinking.

Equipment: Does your school have the equipment needed? If not, can it be purchased or built? (Appendix A lists sources for ordering equipment; Appendix B gives instructions for building equipment.)

Suitability for your facilities: Do you have enough space to accommodate testing? Would you if you tested in smaller groups? Does testing require a track?

Time required for testing: Can the tests be administered to a group, or must they be done individually? Is self-testing possible? Is recording scores difficult? Could time be reduced if you had assistants? Will it take extra training time to teach students the protocol?

Difficulty in explaining or practicing the tests: Are the testing instructions complicated? Do you have to set up special equipment to practice?

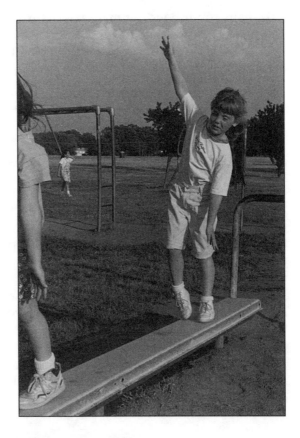

Support Materials and Services

Today's test batteries may come with a wide assortment of support materials.

Manuals: The manual should include a detailed definition of fitness, test standards and an explanation of how they were set, and clear instructions for administering all tests.

Computer software: Computer programs usually analyze test data and print out individual test results. Most test packages have software for both IBM and Apple computers.

Curriculum materials: Materials can include anything from short pamphlets to full-sized books and may also be accompanied by posters and charts.

Instructional videos: Videos may either instruct testers on how to administer the test or teach students about physical fitness.

Knowledge tests: If you teach the basics about physical fitness to your students, such tests allow you to assess how much your students have learned.

Awards: Many testing programs offer awards to be given to students who achieve certain standards of performance. These may be patches, certificates, stickers, T-shirts, and many other low-cost items, often carrying the logo of the testing program.

Teacher incentive program: A few testing programs offer incentive gifts such as a key chain, cap, pen, or mug to teachers who participate in their programs.

To help you use testing materials, to answer questions about testing, and to assist with those inevitable glitches in installing and using software, many test developers also now offer customer service. It's usually available on a telephone helpline, which may or may not be a toll-free number.

Cost

Most schools have to be more careful than ever with their spending, so you're probably looking for the most cost-efficient way to do fitness testing. Luckily, some components cost little or nothing.

It's also important, though, to base your choice not only on how much you get for your money but also on whether you'll use the tests. If they don't measure your program objectives, or if the additional materials included in the test package aren't really helpful in your program, the least expensive option may not be the best. Prices for some of the major test batteries and their components are listed in chapter 3.

When considering costs, be sure to think about any continuing expenses for testing beyond the initial purchase. Will you have to buy score sheets each time you test? Curriculum materials? Awards? Additional or replacement equipment?

Each test package differs, so choose among them according to your needs and the cost involved. In the next chapter we'll describe the contents of each of six major test batteries.

Measurement Capabilities of Tests

A final consideration in choosing a test battery is the quality of the tests themselves: How well do they measure what they're supposed to measure? The quality of test batteries and tests can be evaluated on three characteristics: validity, reliability, and objectivity.

Validity is the underlying worth of the test's measurements. Does the test in fact measure what it is intended to? For example, what scientific evidence supports the use of a distance run as a measure of cardiorespiratory function or aerobic capacity?

Reliability is how consistently the test measures performance. Is a student who scores 50 on a test today likely to earn a similar score several days later?

Objectivity is the accuracy of the scoring scheme for the test. For instance, if triceps skinfold thickness of a student was measured twice by two different testers, would they arrive at the same measurement?

Let's go into each of these characteristics in more depth.

Validity

Validity is the most important aspect of a test. A test that doesn't carry out its intended purpose isn't very useful. When you evaluate a fitness test battery answer these questions:

1. How valid is the test battery as a whole? Does it reflect a sound definition of physical fitness, one based on scientific research?

2. How valid is each test in the battery?
3. How valid is the performance standard for each test? It's especially important to check criterion-referenced standards to know how the standards were determined.

Validity is usually reported using a statistic known as a *correlation coefficient* that represents the strength of the relationship between two variables, usually the results of two tests. The results of the test in the fitness battery are compared with those of the best possible direct measure of the fitness component being tested. The relationship is calculated using a statistical formula.

One example would be the validity of distance run scores for measuring cardiorespiratory fitness. The scores from the distance run have been compared with those from a maximum stress test on a treadmill, a test that directly measures cardiorespiratory fitness. Few of us could afford the equipment and expertise to put all of our students through a maximum stress test, so instead we use the distance run as a more practical assessment tool. Because there is a fairly strong correlation between the results of the two tests, the distance run is a valid test.

A strong correlation is indicated by a high correlation coefficient. Coefficients range from −1.00 to +1.00, and an acceptable coefficient for validity would be ±.80 or higher. Coefficients can be positive or negative. In fact, the correlation between a timed distance run and maximal oxygen uptake is negative. As people run the distance in a shorter time, their maximum oxygen uptake increases. One measure goes down while the other goes up.

But how do we judge tests that directly measure fitness components? A maximum stress test on a treadmill cannot be validated statistically, but we can use a logical analysis. As the workload on the treadmill increases, the subject's maximal oxygen uptake increases (up to a point). When workload increases and maximal oxygen uptake levels off, the subject has reached maximum aerobic capacity. The stress test meets logical analysis; it has *logical validity*.

Test batteries can only be judged by logical validity: Do the tests in the battery fit the definition of physical fitness put forth by the test developer? That definition should be precise, so it is clear to you how the components of fitness in the tests grow out of that definition.

The validity of standards is more difficult to assess. Norm-referenced standards are based on actual scores, so there isn't much question about how they were chosen. Criterion-based standards are supposed to be based on scientific evidence, but unfortunately not enough work has yet been done to support them all. Only the one-mile walk/run and the sum of skinfolds test have sufficient supporting data. As time goes by we hope to see more work done to justify criterion-based standards.

Reliability

Reliability is the consistency with which a student would achieve the same score if the test were taken on different days. Without reliability, we could have no confidence that the score was a stable representation of the child's level of fitness.

Most physical fitness items are highly reliable when students perform their best. Tests requiring a maximal effort can have high reliability coefficients, above .80 and even into the .90s. Not all children, however, have the discipline and tolerance for discomfort to perform at their maximum, which may reduce the reliability of their scores.

Reliability may also be lowered if students don't know how to perform a test. In such a situation they must focus on learning to do the task rather than giving it their all. Then, once they have learned it, their scores may improve on subsequent tests, thus making the scores less reliable.

Children's emotional states can affect reliability as well. Students who are depressed, sad, tired, or stressed may perform below their ability.

Objectivity

Objectivity can have as much to do with the testers as it does with the test itself. Testers must know the proper procedures thoroughly if they are to score in the same manner each time. However, some tests are easier to judge than others.

A distance test run, for example, is easy to score objectively. As long as the stopwatch is started when the signal is given and stopped when the student crosses the finish line, anyone reading the stopwatch would record the same information. As long as there's no recording error, the score is quite objective.

A sit-up test is more difficult to score objectively. It may seem easy at first—all you do is count the number of sit-ups, right?—but only properly executed sit-ups should be counted. It's difficult to make this judgment, and it's usually impossible to watch every single sit-up made by every child. One way to improve this situation is to train students to do the sit-ups correctly before testing, resulting in fewer improperly executed sit-ups. The same applies to pull-ups.

For skinfold measurement, the key to acceptable objectivity rests with the tester. The tester should practice measuring skinfolds many times before actually testing students. Some experienced testers recommend taking as many as 100 practice skinfold measurements in advance.

Checklist for Choosing a Testing Program

If you've read this far, you now have some solid criteria for choosing a test battery. We've discussed program philosophy, practical considerations, and test quality. To help you select a testing program, we've consolidated all these criteria in the following checklist. Use it as you examine the six testing programs described in the next chapter, or copy it as a guide for judging other test programs in which you are interested.

TESTING PROGRAM CHECKLIST

Program Philosophy

    ✓ Are standards norm-based or criterion-based?

    ✓ Are tests health-related or performance-related?

Practical Considerations

✓ Are all tests appropriate for your students? Consider their age, gender, culture, and disabilities.

✓ Are the tests easy to administer? What about equipment needed, suitability for your facility, time required for testing, and difficulty of explaining or practicing the tests?

✓ What support materials does this battery offer? What quality are the manuals, computer software, instructional videos, curriculum materials, knowledge tests, awards, teacher incentives, and phone helpline?

✓ What will it cost to buy this battery? What will it cost to use it regularly if disposable materials are needed (scoring sheets, computer printout forms, booklets, awards, etc.)?

Measurement Capabilities

✓ For each test in the battery, what is its validity, reliability, and objectivity?

✓ Is the battery logically valid?

✓ Are the standards valid?

Summary

- Three criteria for selecting a test battery are your philosophy of fitness education, the practical aspects of the battery's use, and the validity, reliability, and objectivity of the tests and test battery.
- Norm-referenced standards represent how a group of students, usually a nationwide representative group, performed on a test. They often are represented as percentiles. Norms
  - depend on the set of scores used to establish them,
  - are meant to be used for interpreting individual scores only, not group scores, and
  - can create unrealistic expectations for student performance.
- Criterion-referenced standards are based on research done to set the minimum level of fitness for good health. To have a criterion-referenced standard, a test must measure some aspect of health. Criterion-referenced standards
  - are not yet proven to be accurate,
  - don't always motivate highly fit students, and
  - are subject to examination of their validity and reliability.
- Criterion-referenced standards are best as the primary standard for individuals, but norms are useful for comparing students with others across the country and for recognizing high levels of achievement.
- The choice of health-related or performance-related tests depends on whether you want to measure for health or for high achievement. In general, health-related tests have criterion-referenced standards, and performance-related tests have norm-referenced standards.

- The suitability of a test battery for your class depends on the battery's appropriateness for your students, ease of administration, support materials and service, and cost.
- The quality of a test battery is measured by its tests' validity, reliability, and objectivity.
- Validity is a measure of how well a test measures what it is intended to measure. High test validity is shown by a high correlation coefficient between the most direct measure of a variable and the test, preferably at least ±.80. (Direct measurements are judged by logical validity.) Test batteries can be judged only by logical validity, and criterion-based standards by research data.
- Reliability, a measure of how consistently a test measures performance, is best for tests that require a maximal effort. Reliability may be lowered if students aren't familiar with test protocols or if they are in emotionally negative states.
- Objectivity is a measure of whether multiple testers arrive at the same score. Test results that can be measured mechanically, such as time or number of laps, are most objective. Results that require the tester to use judgment are less objective.

References

AAHPER. (1976). *Youth fitness test.* Washington, DC: Author.

Koebel, C.I., Swank, A.M., & Swinburne, L. (1992). Fitness testing in children: A comparison between PCPFS and AAHPERD standards. *Journal of Applied Sport Science Research,* **6**(2), 107-114.

President's Council on Physical Fitness and Sports (PCPFS). (1989). *President's Challenge Physical Fitness Program.* Washington, DC: Author.

Reiff, G.G., Dixon, W.R., Jacoby, D., Ye, G.X., Spain, C.G., & Hunsicker, P.A. (1985). *National school population fitness survey* (Research Project 282-84-0086). Washington, DC: The President's Council on Physical Fitness and Sports.

Ross, J.G., & Gilbert, G.G. (1985). The national children and youth fitness study: A summary of findings. *Journal of Physical Education, Recreation and Dance.* **56**, 45-50.

Ross, J.G., & Pate, R.R. (1987). The national children and youth fitness study II: A summary of findings. *Journal of Physical Education, Recreation and Dance.* **58**, 51-61.

Safrit, M.J. (1990). *An introduction to measurement in physical education and exercise science* (2nd ed.). St. Louis: Times Mirror/Mosby.

Spray, J.A. (1977). Interpreting group or class performances using AAHPER Youth Fitness Test norms. *Journal of Physical Education and Recreation,* **48**, 56-57.

CHAPTER 3

The Physical Fitness Testing Programs

Now that we've discussed how to choose a testing program, let's examine some of the major programs used in the United States today. You probably have at least heard of most of them, and you may have used one or more in your teaching.

The testing programs described in this chapter are these:

1. AAHPERD Physical Best Program
2. Chrysler Fund/AAU Physical Fitness Program
3. Prudential FITNESSGRAM
4. President's Challenge Physical Fitness Program
5. YMCA Youth Fitness Test
6. National Youth Physical Fitness Program

For each of these testing programs we present the following information:

- *Test sponsor and developer:* Who supports the test program? Who developed it?

- *Target population:* For what age range is the test appropriate? Can the test be modified for use with children with disabilities?

- *Definition of fitness:* How does this test define fitness? What components of fitness are included?

- *Tests:* What tests are included in the test battery? (All tests will be described in more detail in chapter 4.)

- *Standards and award system:* What standards are provided? Is there an award system? If so, what are the criteria for winning awards?

- *Materials:* What is included in the testing package? How can materials be obtained? What do they cost?

- *Software:* If software is available, what does it do? What hardware does it require? What does it cost? How easy is it to install and use?

You will find much of this information summarized in tables at the end of this chapter so you can easily compare the test programs.

The information in this chapter is current as the book is being written, but changes occur quickly in the area of testing. The FITNESSGRAM program has recently undergone major revisions, and the AAU program also has been altered. A major change that occurred while this book was being written was the agreement between the Cooper Institute for Aerobics Research (the developers of FITNESSGRAM) and AAHPERD (the developers of the Physical Best test battery) to join forces. As a result of their 5-year agreement, beginning in December 1993, AAHPERD dropped Physical Best as its test and adopted FITNESSGRAM. During 1994 both organizations will continue to offer both their award systems as they work out a new joint award system. The educational materials from both programs will be available from either organization through a joint order form. Physical Best software is no longer available.

AAHPERD Physical Best Program

Test Sponsor and Developer

American Alliance for Health, Physical Education, Recreation and Dance (AAHPERD)

Target Population

Ages 5 to 18. Use with special populations is recommended and a supplement for special populations is to be released in August 1994.

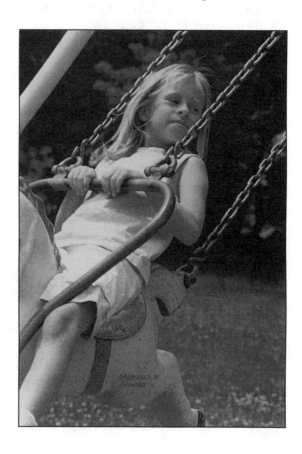

Definition of Fitness

Physical fitness is defined as "a physical state of well-being that allows people to (1) perform daily activities with vigor; (2) reduce their risk of health problems related to lack of exercise; and (3) establish a fitness base for participation in a variety of physical activities" (McSwegin, Pemberton, Petray, & Going, 1989, p. 1).

Tests

The Physical Best test battery was withdrawn from use by AAHPERD in December of 1993 and replaced by FITNESSGRAM. However, the award system will remain in effect through 1994 until a new one is established. The battery's five tests are shown in Table 3.1.

Standards and Award System

The award system presented here may change by the end of 1994 because of the joint agreement between AAHPERD and the Cooper Institute for Aerobics Research. Criterion-referenced standards are presented for each test. No tables of norms are included in the program guide, but normative data are available from the National Children and Youth Fitness I and II studies. Both sets of data appear in Appendix C.

The award system, called the American Alliance Physical Best Recognition System (AAHPERD, 1988), includes three types of awards:

- The Fitness Activity Award is given to recognize participation in appropriate physical activity outside of class. To win this award, a child must maintain a log of physical fitness activities.
- The Fitness Goals Award is presented for attaining individual fitness goals developed by the child with the help of a physical education teacher.

Table 3.1   AAHPERD Physical Best Test Battery

Item	Component of fitness
One-mile walk/run (or any running test 6 min or longer)	Aerobic capacity
Sum of tricep and calf skinfolds (or sum of tricep and subscapular skinfolds or body mass index)	Body composition
Sit-and-reach test	Flexibility
Modified sit-ups test	Muscular strength and endurance
Pull-ups	Muscular strength and endurance

- The Health Fitness Award recognizes a child for achieving health fitness standards. To receive this award, the child must attain the minimum acceptable level of fitness on all tests.

Badges (patches) and certificates are available for each award level.

Materials

The following materials are packaged into an Educational Kit:

- An *Instructor's Guide*, introducing the test battery and the key program components
- Teaching Idea Cards, which cover information on health-related fitness concepts (Each card contains the definition of a fitness concept, an activity to reinforce the concept, and additional suggestions for learning center activities. See Figure 3.1 for a sample Teaching Idea Card.)
- Samples of a class record, individual contract, activity log, and individual report card for testing
- A poster
- Information on using the award system

Educational Kits are available for Grades K to 6 and 6 to 12. Tests are the same for both, but the Teaching Idea Cards differ. If your sixth-grade class is part of an elementary school, order the K-to-6 kit; if the class is part of a middle school, choose the 6-to-12 kit. The Educational Kit costs $37.95; the kit and software, sold as an Educational Pack, are $62.95.

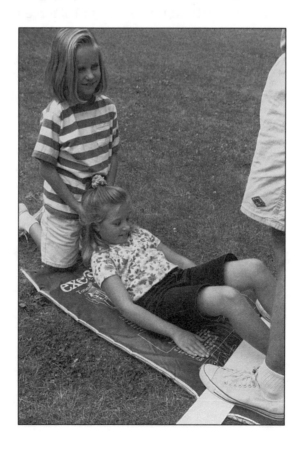

Section II, K-3

Idea 1: Aerobic Endurance Component

Concept: Define aerobic endurance

K-3: Aerobic endurance is using your heart, lungs, and muscles to do exercise over a long period of time. To explain this concept, tell the students that the body is like a car. The heart, lungs, and muscles are like the fuel lines, motor, and wheels of your car. Fuel is pumped in the motor and the fuel lines deliver gasoline so the wheels can spin and move. The heart and lungs act as a motor and deliver fuel (oxygen) to the muscle, which, like the wheels of the car, move. Having aerobic endurance will help keep you from "running out of gas."

Activity: Moving across America

Choose a movement, such as walking, wogging (combination of walking and jogging), jogging, or running. Have the students participate in this activity for a certain amount of time each class period. Begin the duration of this activity at a low level, 2 to 3 min. Then increase the duration over time. Compute the mileage the entire class does over each class period as well as over an extended period of time. Chart the mileage each day or week on a map of your state or the country.

Learning center suggestion

Discuss various forms of aerobic endurance activities with the students. Ask them to think of games they play that are aerobic in nature. Which makes them breathe harder than usual? Which makes their hearts beat faster? Which uses large muscles in their legs, arms, and bodies? Which can be played nonstop?

Figure 3.1 Sample teaching idea card.
Note. from *Physical Best* by American Alliance for Health, Physical Education, Recreation and Dance, 1988, Reston, VA: Author. Copyright 1988 by American Alliance for Health, Physical Education, Recreation and Dance. Reprinted with permission from American Alliance for Health, Physical Education, Recreation and Dance.

Additional copies of the activity log, contracts, and report cards are available in packs of 30. The activity logs and contracts are $5, and the report cards are $3.50. Additional copies of the *Instructor's Guide* can be purchased for $6.95; additional posters are $10 each. Official awards are $1.75 each for badges and $.35 each for certificates. Additional award materials such as T-shirts, pins, shoelaces, pencils, and stickers can be ordered separately, as can testing equipment.

Two videos also can be purchased. *Physical Best: Integrating Concepts With Activities* ($19.95) depicts activities that integrate fitness concepts into sports and games. This video is available in two versions, one for Grades K to 6 and the other for Grades 6 to 12. *Measuring Body Fat Using Skinfolds* ($29.95) is instructional, demonstrating appropriate skinfold measurement techniques.

All materials, including the software described next, are available from the following address:

AAHPERD Publications
P. O. Box 704
Waldorf, MD 20604
800-321-0789

For answers to questions about the program, call the Physical Best office at 703-476-3426.

Software

Software for the Physical Best test is no longer available. At the time of writing the toll-free helpline for software was going to operate until at least September 1994 and longer if usage warranted. The helpline will be answered by a machine during the day. Calls are promptly returned within 24 hours.

> Available in Apple or IBM, 3-1/2 in. and 5-1/4 in. disks. Comes with a manual. Cost is $34.95 if purchased separately from the Educational Pack.

Physical Best Software II consists of two disks. The 5-1/4 in. disks can hold 1,500 student records; the 3-1/2 in. disks hold 6,000 records.

Hardware requirements are as follows:

- Apple: IIe, IIc, GS, or Apple compatible, with 128k and ProDOS
- IBM: PC, PS 2, XT, AT, or IBM compatible, with 256k and a minimum of DOS 2.1

Two drives are required, and a hard disk may be used, but is not necessary. Permissible types of printers are not mentioned in the manual.

For a card reader to record test scores you must purchase either an OMR 1000 Manual Feed ($899) or an OMR 200 High Speed Autofeed ($1,366). Scan cards are available from the same address as the software (250 double-sided cards hold 500 records for $32).

The main menu includes these options:

- Student data: Input, review, or update student information data screens.

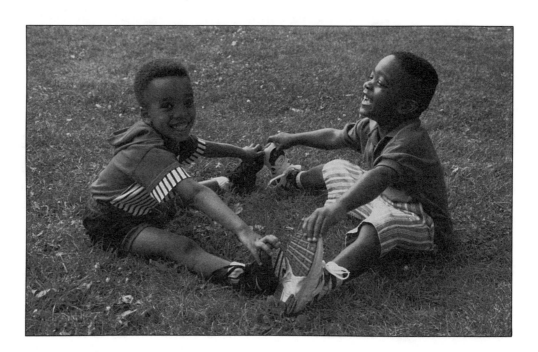

- Create reports: Display or print 16 reports (such as an individual student's performance, all of the students performing to standards, etc.).
- Goal options: Review and create goals.
- Consolidations: Consolidate data (calculate statistics analyses) according to grade, school, district, state, and nation.
- Setup: Enter names of instructors and school or organization on the program disk.

Not all menu functions are currently available. High-resolution graphics are used throughout the program.

The user's manual is easy to read and helpful, but the program has some "bugs" that make it difficult to use. A toll-free helpline for software is available from 8:00 p.m. to 5:00 p.m. daily. A staff member may answer, machine-recorded calls will be returned.

Chrysler Fund/AAU Physical Fitness Program

Test Sponsor and Developer

Chrysler Fund/Amateur Athletic Union (AAU)

Target Population

Ages 6 to 17. The AAU program suggests specific test modifications, has a special award system, and gives general guidelines for exercise programs for children with disabilities. Camps and scout groups use it as well as schools.

Definition of Fitness

Physical fitness is "made up of several specific dimensions, each of which must be developed individually. These include strength, muscular endurance, cardiorespiratory endurance and flexibility. These cannot be measured by a single test item, nor will excellence in one category compensate for deficiencies in another" (Chrysler Fund/Amateur Athletic Union, 1993-94, p. 12).

The AAU Physical Fitness Program emphasizes fitness literacy, which is defined as "a process that involves physiological and cognitive adaptation" (Benham, 1988, p. 7). "A child attains fitness literacy by experiencing change in his or her personal fitness and learning essential knowledge associated with physical fitness" (Updyke, 1987, p. 1). Essential knowledge includes understanding risk factors associated with disease, in particular, physical inactivity, and knowing the rationale for developing and maintaining cardio-respiratory endurance, flexibility, and muscular strength and endurance. Knowing exercise prescription is also important. Finally, children should understand how fitness is influenced by heredity, by their initial levels of fitness, and by their developmental stages (Benham, 1988).

Tests

The test battery consists of four required tests and seven optional ones. They are listed in Table 3.2.

The distances selected for the endurance run vary with student's ages: 1/4 mi for ages 6 to 7, 1/2 mi for ages 8 to 9, 3/4 mi for ages 10 to 11, and 1 mi for ages 12 and over. The pull-ups and flexed arm hang have been modified to permit participants to use a grip that is either toward the body or away from the body.

All required tests are health-related, but some of the optional tests are for motor skills. The test developers distinguish between physical fitness and motor skill: "Unlike physical fitness, skill may be retained at reasonably high levels even without regular practice. Both physical fitness and motor skills are important in physical performance, but they are developed in different ways. In general, physical fitness is *earned*—skill is *learned*" (Chryser Fund/AAU, 1993-94, p. 2).

Standards and Award System

Norm-referenced standards are presented for each test. The normative data provided by the test developer are calculated from test scores submitted by teachers on a voluntary basis, so the norms may not be representative of American children and youth across the country.

Three awards may be given in this program:

- The Certificate of Outstanding Performance for children who score at the 80th percentile or higher on all five tests
- The Certificate of Attainment for children who score from the 45th to the 79th percentile on all five tests (possibly higher on some)
- The Certificate of Participation for children who score below the 45th percentile on at least one test

Table 3.2   AAU Test Battery

Item	Component of fitness
Required tests	
Endurance run	Cardiorespiratory endurance
Bent-knee sit-ups	Trunk strength and endurance
Sit-and-reach test	Flexibility in hamstrings and low back
Pull-ups*	
Flexed arm hang**	Upper-body strength and endurance
Optional tests	
Hoosier endurance run	Cardiorespiratory endurance
Standing long jump	Leg strength; efficiency of body mass
Isometric push-ups	Upper-body static endurance
Modified push-ups (girls)	Upper-body strength and endurance
Phantom chair	Static leg endurance
Shuttle run	Agility and quickness
Sprints	Speed, quickness, and anaerobic ability

*Required for Outstanding award level.
**Required for Attainment and Participation award levels.

Materials

The heart of the AAU Physical Fitness Program is a brochure called a *Testing Packet*. It includes test protocols, scoring sheets and norms, the award system, and information on the other materials available. The *Testing Packet* and a brochure called *Special Test Tips*, for students with special needs, are free. *Special Test Tips* includes general test modifications, an award system, references, and addresses for associations with fitness and sport information. It also contains general guidelines for exercise programs for children with

Pulmonary diseases	Sensory impairments
Physical disabilities	Mental retardation
Cardiac conditions	Autism
Endocrine diseases	Emotional and social
AIDS	impairments
Nutritional diseases	Severe impairments
Neuromuscular diseases	

Many other materials are available at low cost. They include the following:

- Jungle animal poster series promoting exercise (four fitness education posters for $2 each or $7 for all four)
- Motivational poster series (five posters, one of which shows award performance criteria, for $1 each or $4 for all five)
- *Fitness Curriculum*, a teacher's manual and activity cards ($12)
- *Nutrition Curriculum*, a teacher's manual to be used cooperatively by the classroom teacher and physical education teacher ($12)
- *Home Fitness Curriculum*, a module designed to promote the development and maintenance of physical fitness outside the classroom that involves other family members ($12)
- *Fitness Fanfare*, a two-part fitness-testing video. The motivational part is a storyline about members of a high-school band who need to be physically fit to participate in band activities; the instructional part consists of demonstrations of all tests ($7 rental fee, $29.95 purchase price)
- A slide chart for quickly determining awards criteria ($3)
- Award certificates, which are free if you send in your score sheets ($10 shipping charge for up to 599 awards; $1 for each additional 100)
- A free gift for the instructor who sends in the score sheets

All materials, including the software discussed next, can be ordered from the following address:

Chrysler Fund/AAU Physical Fitness Program
Poplars Building
Bloomington, IN 47405
800-258-5497

A toll-free helpline is available from 9 a.m. to 5 p.m. daily.

Software

> Available in Apple, Macintosh, and IBM 3-1/2 in. and 5-1/4 in. disks. Cost is $15.

The AAU Physical Fitness Program software package consists of one or two disks and a three-page set of instructions. Hardware requirements are these:

- Any Apple or Apple-compatible computer with 128k, an 80-column card, and a printer
- Any Macintosh or Macintosh-compatible computer with system version 6.0 or above and a printer
- Any IBM or IBM-compatible computer with 256k and a printer

This software can score between 500 and 1,000 student records.

The main menu offers the following options for Apple and IBM:

- Record sheet: Enter, revise, or print participant records.
- Award summary profile: Display number of awards and generate summary form.
- Percentile profile: Calculate percentiles for individuals or groups.
- Utilities: Generate percentage for each AAU test item and allow copying of participants to a new or different group.
- Exit this program: Return user to current operating system.

The main choices for Macintosh include these:

- File: Access and print record sheet; print group roster; view and print award summary form, individual or group profiles (which can be further broken down into age or sex groupings); and print complete percentile table.
- Score: Enter group information; add, edit, or delete group names; edit individuals sequentially or randomly; view record sheet and group roster; and transfer individuals to another or different group.
- Awards: View, edit, and clear school information; provide part of optional AAU questionnaire information.
- Profiles: View individual and group percentile profiles and raw scores.

This program is user-friendly and easy to use. It is menu-driven and has clear instructions that are easy to follow. If you should have problems, a phone helpline is available daily. When we called, we received prompt and courteous answers to our questions. Upon purchasing the software, you are automatically registered to receive updated software materials at no additional cost.

Prudential FITNESSGRAM

Test Sponsor and Developer

The Prudential Insurance Company and the Cooper Institute for Aerobics Research

Target Population

Ages 5 to 17+. Modifications of FITNESSGRAM for special populations, such as the use of a swimming test instead of a distance run or the use of a shorter distance run for younger children, appear in section five of the test administration manual. You can record modified test results on a noncomputerized form, which allows teachers to give any test and use their own standards.

Definition of Fitness

The Prudential FITNESSGRAM handbook lists three components of health-related physical fitness that correspond to overall health status and optimal function: aerobic capacity, body composition, and muscle strength, endurance, and flexibility. Those components are defined here:

> Aerobic capacity relative to body weight is considered to be the best indicator of a person's overall cardiorespiratory capacity. Acceptable levels of aerobic capacity are associated with a reduced risk of high blood pressure, coronary heart disease, obesity, diabetes, some forms of cancer and other health problems. (p. 8)

> Body composition . . . provide[s] an estimation of the percent of a student's weight that is fat in contrast to fat free body mass (muscles, bones, organs). Maintaining appropriate body composition is vital in preventing the onset of obesity, which is associated with increased risk of coronary heart disease, stroke, and diabetes. (p. 13)

> It is . . . important to have strong muscles that can work forcefully and/or over a period of time and also be adequately flexible to allow full range of motion at the joint. Musculoskeletal injuries are many times the result of imbalance at a specific joint; the muscles on one side may be much stronger than the opposition muscles or may have inadequate flexibility to allow complete motion or sudden motion to appear. (p. 17)

Tests

If you are familiar with versions of FITNESSGRAM prior to fall 1992, this current version is markedly different. The tests are shown in Table 3.3.

This test battery provides several tests to measure many of the components of health-related fitness. You can choose between them or use the recommended test. Under Aerobic Capacity, the PACER test, a multistage 20-m shuttle run, is recommended for children in Grades K to 2. This test battery was adopted by AAHPERD in December 1993 as a replacement for the Physical Best test battery.

Standards and Award System

The award system presented here may change by the end of 1994. A new award system may result from the joint agreement between AAHPERD and the Cooper Institute for Aerobics Research.

Criterion-referenced standards are presented in two levels, Good and Better, that fall within the Healthy Fitness Zone (see Appendix D). A performance below the Good standard is classified as falling into the Needs Improvement Zone. Scores above Better are acknowledged, but not viewed as essential. No norm-referenced standards are included.

Table 3.3 Prudential FITNESSGRAM Test Battery

Item	Component of fitness
Aerobic capacity One-mile walk/run* The PACER	Aerobic capacity
Muscle strength, endurance, and flexibility Curl-ups*	Abdominal strength
90-degree push-ups* Pull-ups Flexed arm hang Modified pull-ups	Upper-body strength
Trunk lift*	Trunk extensor strength and flexibility
Back saver sit-and-reach* Shoulder stretch	Flexibility
Body composition Skinfold measurements* Body mass index	Body composition

*Recommended item used as the default choice on the software.

Several programs are available under the FITNESSGRAM recognition system. The first is the *Get Fit* program for fitness behavior in which children earn special items by participating in a 6-week conditioning program.

It's Your Move! is a second, brand-new recognition program. This program provides children with a booklet from which to choose various physical activities. They must complete 20 activities within 5 to 7 weeks. The children must participate in at least two activities from each of the following six sections: physical fitness testing, home activities, personal activities, school activities, neighborhood activities, and activities with friends. For example, the "Activities to Do by Yourself" section lists activities such as roller skating, riding a bike, and playing hopscotch. A child in Grade K, 1, or 2 would select two activities from the list and participate in each for 10 to 20 min. Students do not receive recognition for test performance, but for sharing FITNESSGRAM results with a parent or guardian and developing a written list of areas needing improvement. The teacher can award a certificate, when the child completes the activities selected from the *It's Your Move!* booklet.

Fit for Life is the third recognition program available. It is for individuals who have displayed commendable exercise behavior outside the school program during a 6-week period. Students can maintain an exercise log for this program or set specific goals or even create a contract. Both children and adults may participate. Reproducible copies of a contract and exercise log are included with the test administration manual.

The final recognition program is *I'm Fit*, which focuses on meeting test standards or improving test scores. Participants (either children or adults) earn recognition by meeting five of the six criterion-referenced standards or by showing improvement in performance on at least two tests.

Materials

This test program includes the following materials:

- A manual describing the test items
- A handbook for teachers
- Forms
- FITNESSGRAM computer printout cards ($22 for 200 or $60 for 600; price includes free software and software manual, test administration manual, and a poster)
- Testing equipment (as part of the special enrollment package or purchased separately)
- *It's Your Move!* sets ($19.55 for a set: 35 activities books and additional items)
- Awards
- Videotape

The manual, *The Prudential FITNESSGRAM Test Administration Manual* (Cooper Institute for Aerobics Research, 1992), is a testing and curriculum guide. It includes sections on physical fitness testing, test administration, modifications for special populations, interpretation of results, fitness programming, and recognition and motivation. An envelope with 14 blackline masters including all program forms accompanies it. The manual is free with a purchase of computer cards or the special enrollment package. Additional copies can be purchased for $10 each or two for $15.

The handbook, *Teaching Strategies for Improving Youth Fitness* (Corbin & Pangrazi, n.d.), describes the Prudential FITNESSGRAM philosophy, and the preparation, administration, and recognition system involved with the test battery. It includes 40 blackline masters for making overheads and handouts, plus excellent resource lists. This book is now out of print, but an updated version will be available in fall 1994.

A special enrollment package is available that includes the test administration and software manuals; computer software; testing tapes and equipment; blackline masters of scoresheets, exercise logs, goals sheets, contracts, certificates, and training heart rate zones; and samples of all recognition items. The cost is $76. Testing tapes and equipment can be purchased separately. The curl-up measuring strip is $.45; skinfold calipers are $4.75; and the PACER tape and lap counter are $10.

It's Your Move! sets, used for the recognition program of the same name, are available for three grade levels: K to 2 (*Hip Hoppers*), 3 to 4 (*Movers & Shakers*), and 5 to 6 (*Slam Jammers*). Each set includes 35 activity booklets, a classroom recognition poster and tracking stickers, and a blackline master for a recognition certificate. Recognition buttons are available separately.

Recognition awards are $.25 each for ribbons, $.25–$.45 each for certificates, and $.35 each for buttons. Other awards such as pencils, stickers, and embroidered emblems are available, as well as additional instructor paraphernalia such as jackets, T-shirts, pins, and shoelaces.

A videotape, *The Prudential FITNESSGRAM Program*, describes the importance of physical fitness and regular physical activity and demonstrates the FITNESSGRAM tests. Prudential insurance agents show the video to agencies interested in adopting the Prudential FITNESSGRAM Program, and it is available only through them.

All materials except the videotape can be ordered from the following address:

The Prudential FITNESSGRAM
12330 Preston Rd.
Dallas, TX 75230
800-635-7050 or
214-701-8001

A toll-free helpline is available from 9:00 a.m. to 5:00 p.m. Monday through Friday.

In the future the educational materials related to FITNESSGRAM will be developed by AAHPERD with input from FITNESSGRAM. For now, all educational materials from either the FITNESSGRAM or Physical Best program can be obtained through either program office.

Software

Available in Apple, Macintosh, and IBM (with or without Windows), 3-1/2 in. or 5-1/4 in. disks. IBM and Macintosh versions come with two manuals; the Apple version comes with one. Cost is free with first purchase of computer forms or the Special Enrollment Package. Additional copies of the computer reference manual are $10 each or 2 for $15.

FITNESSGRAM software consists of a single disk (two for IBM, one of them being for Windows). It requires a computer with a hard disk and at least 640k of memory and will run on the following:

- Apple IIe or GS, ProDOS (Apple IIe version does not contain all test options; a new, complete version will be released in spring 1994)
- Macintosh, Finder or Multifinder
- IBM PC, XT, or PS, MS-DOS (a Windows version is available)

The program works with Epson, IBM, or Panasonic printers or with the Hewlett Packard laser printer, and a new printer can be added.

The program's main menu provides these options:

- File: Change databases, display the current database file name, access the help information, exit.
- Database: Enter information.
- Reports: Access information contained in the database and produce desired reports (such as summary reports for all students or individual students, achievement of standards, etc.).
- Utility: Use general purpose utility functions.

You can enter data through an Opticon II Scantron scanner. The forms for the scanner come 500 to a box and cost $60. The FITNESSGRAM scanner software is included with the program software.

The unique FITNESSGRAM report card that this software generates is helpful in explaining test results to children and their parents. A sample FITNESSGRAM appears in Figure 3.2.

The Prudential FITNESSGRAM program is very easy to use. Installation is straightforward, and a help option is available in the Utility menu that provides assistance for running all the program options. Assistance is available on a phone helpline.

Besides the computer reference manual, an additional simplified manual called *Quickstart* helps you get around in the FITNESSGRAM program. *Quickstart* is available for IBM and Macintosh hardware, and an Apple version was released in spring of 1994.

The FITNESSGRAM program is sophisticated. For example, in the Windows version, once the program has been installed, it automatically sets up a FIT-NESSGRAM icon for accessing the program. You can copy relevant scores and class rosters from the previous software directly to the data disk generated by the new software. You can also copy an ASCII version of class rosters to the new FITNESSGRAM data disk.

President's Challenge Physical Fitness Program

Test Sponsor and Developer

The President's Council on Physical Fitness and Sports (PCPFS)

Target Population

Ages 6 to 17. The President's Challenge program allows modifications or substitutions for battery tests for children with special needs, but does not suggest specific ones. Such changes are based on the judgment of qualified instructors who follow the criteria stated in the test booklet.

Definition of Fitness

Physical fitness is defined as follows:

> Being physically fit means having the energy and strength to perform daily activities vigorously and alertly without getting "run down," and having energy left over to enjoy leisure-time activities or meet emergency demands. When you are physically fit, your heart, lungs, and muscles are strong and your body is firm and flexible. Your weight and body fat are within a desirable range. (PCPFS, 1993a, p. 6)

Three components of fitness are identified in this program: endurance (cardio-respiratory and muscular), strength, and flexibility.

- Endurance is defined as "the ability to keep moving for long periods of time" (PCPFS, 1993a, p. 7).
- Strength is defined as "how much force you can exert with your muscles" (PCPFS, 1993a, p. 8).

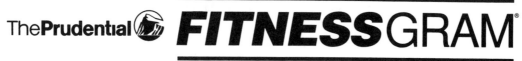

The Prudential FITNESSGRAM®

COMMITTED TO HEALTH RELATED FITNESS

Joe Jogger
Central Jr. High School
Central I. S. D.

Instructor: **Mr. James**
Grade: **06**   Period: **05**   Age: **13**

Test Date	Height	Weight
MO - YR	FT - IN	LBS
10.92	5.00	101
05.93	5.03	110

AEROBIC CAPACITY

HEALTHY FITNESS ZONE

One Mile Walk/Run

Needs Improvement	Good	Better
*************************		
10:00		07:30

VO₂max — VO_{2max} — Indicates ability to use oxygen. Expressed as ml of oxygen per kg body weight per minute. Healthy Fitness Zone = 35+ for girls & 42+ for boys.

	Current	Past
min:sec	9:01	9:12
ml/kg/min	47	47

MUSCLE STRENGTH, ENDURANCE & FLEXIBLITY

HEALTHY FITNESS ZONE

Curl-up (Abdominal)

Needs Improvement	Good	Better
*******		
21		40

# performed	
12	10

Push-up (Upper Body)

Needs Improvement	Good	Better
12		25

# performed	
27	20

Trunk Lift (Trunk Extension)

Needs Improvement	Good	Better
9		12

Inches	
10	10

The test of flexibility is optional. If given, it is scored pass or fail and is performed on the right and left.

Test given: **Back Saver Sit-and-Reach**

Right	P
Left	P

BODY COMPOSITION

HEALTHY FITNESS ZONE

Percent Body Fat

Needs Improvement	Good	Better
25.0		10.0

% Fat	
25.9	31.1

You can improve your abdominal strength with curl-ups 2 to 4 times a week. Remember your knees are bent and no one holds your feet.

Your upper body strength was very good. Try to maintain your fitness by doing strengthening activities at least 2 or 3 times each week.

To improve your body composition, Joe, extend the length of vigorous activity each day and follow a balanced nutritional program, eating more fruits and vegetables and fewer fats and sugars. Improving body composition may also help improve your other fitness scores.

Your aerobic capacity is in the Healthy Fitness Zone. Maintain your fitness by doing 20 – 30 minutes of vigorous activity at least 3 or 4 times each week.

To parent or guardian: *The Prudential FITNESSGRAM is a valuable tool in assessing a young person's fitness level. The area of the bar highlighted in yellow indicates the "healthy fitness zone." All children should strive to maintain levels of fitness within the "healthy fitness zone" or above. By maintaining a healthy fitness level for these areas of fitness your child may have a reduced risk for developing heart disease, obesity or low back pain. Some children may have personal interests that require higher levels of fitness (e.g. athletes).*

Recommended activities for improving fitness are based on each individual's test performance. Ask your child to demonstrate each test item for you. Some teachers may stop the test when performance equals the upper limit of the "healthy fitness zone" rather than requiring a maximal effort.

Developing good exercise habits is important to maintaining lifelong health. You can help your son or daughter develop these habits by encouraging regular participation in physical activity.

© 1992 The Cooper Institute for Aerobics Research

Developed by
The Cooper Institute
for Aerobics Research
Dallas, Texas

Sponsored by
The Prudential
Insurance Company
of America

Figure 3.2   Sample FITNESSGRAM.
Note. From Prudential FITNESSGRAM. Copyright 1992 by the Cooper Institute for Aerobics Research^MM. Reprinted with permission from Cooper Institute for Aerobics Research, Dallas, TX.

- Flexibility is defined as "[being able to] move your muscles and joints through their 'full range of motion'" (PCPFS, 1993a, p. 8).

The program mentions speed, agility, and coordination as additional factors affecting fitness and discusses body composition, but does not include it as part of the test battery. According to the *Get Fit!* booklet (PCPFS, 1993a), children who want to know whether their body composition is good should ask a physical education or health teacher or a fitness instructor to measure percent body fat.

Tests

The tests for the President's Challenge test battery appear in Table 3.4.

The sit-and-reach is measured in centimeters using a sit-and-reach box; the V-sit reach is measured in inches.

Standards and Award System

Norm-referenced standards are used for the President's Challenge Physical Fitness Test. Three levels of awards are given based on the test standards:

- The Presidential Physical Fitness Award for scoring at or above the 85th percentile on all five tests
- The National Physical Fitness Award for scoring at or above the 50th percentile on all five tests
- The Participant Physical Fitness Award for scoring below the 50th percentile on one or more tests

At each level, the award includes a certificate and/or an emblem (patch); other award options also are available.

All three awards are also available to children with special needs if they perform at a level equivalent to a Presidential, National, or Participant level of performance for a boy or girl this age with this condition using the same or modified tests. The individual instructor determines equivalency.

A Presidential Instructor Emblem and wearing apparel are available to instructors whose students qualify for awards. In addition, the State Champion Award recognizes the three top schools in each state, by enrollment, with the

Table 3.4   President's Challenge Test Battery

Item	Component of fitness
Curl-ups	Abdominal strength and endurance
Pull-ups	Upper-body strength and endurance
Flexed arm hang*	Upper-body strength and endurance
One-mile walk/run	Cardiorespiratory endurance
V-sit reach or sit-and-reach	Low back and hamstring flexibility
Shuttle run	Leg strength, agility, endurance, and power

*Alternative test to pull-ups for earning the National or Participant Physical Fitness Award.

highest number of students achieving the Presidential Physical Fitness Award (the three enrollment categories are 50-100 students, 101-500, and above 500). The winning school receives a special certificate and nationwide publicity, and each student gets a certificate and emblem. The school must complete a special entry form from the program packet to be considered, but there is no cost for involvement in the State Champion Award program.

Materials

Materials available for the President's Challenge Physical Fitness Program include the following:

- The *Get Fit!* booklet for students (PCPFS, 1993a), which defines and discusses the major components of fitness and presents warm-up exercises and exercises for each component. A short 10-item fitness quiz ends the booklet.
- *The President's Challenge Physical Fitness Packet* (PCPFS, 1993b), which describes the awards criteria and program (including those for children with special needs), instructions for the tests, and order forms for awards and related items. A poster and a single copy of *Get Fit!* are also included.
- A monograph describing the results of the recent survey of youth fitness conducted by the President's Council on Physical Fitness and Sports, which contains the national norms.
- Awards.

All of these materials except the monograph and the awards are free. Awards range from $.20 to $.50 for each certificate to $.50 to $1.25 for each emblem. The Presidential Instructor Emblem is $1.50 and you can purchase other items such as decals, pins, bumper stickers, and magnets.

All materials can be ordered at this address:

> PCPFS
> 701 Pennsylvania Ave, NW, Suite 250
> Washington, DC 20004

All materials except for the monograph also may be obtained from the following address:

> President's Challenge
> Poplars Research Center
> 400 E. Seventh St.
> Bloomington, IN 47405
> 800-258-8146

Software

> Available in Apple and IBM. Comes with a manual. Cost is $100.

Private vendors developed the software available for the President's Challenge Test. The Council has not reviewed this software.

The President's Challenge software consists of two disks (one for backup). It requires the following hardware:

- Apple II+, IIe, IIc, IIGS with 64k
- IBM PC or Tandy 1000 or a compatible with 264k with a color graphics adapter

Acceptable types of printers are not specified, although the software has a menu for configuring a printer. An Apple disk holds 35 files, 50 students per file; an IBM disk holds 77 files, 50 students per file.

The program is menu-driven and consists of several menu options:

- Main menu: Edit names and scores, print records, delete files, edit norm tables, and quit.
- Create data disks: Store records.
- Copy data disks: Copy information from disks.
- Edit norm tables: Select tests currently being used and modify the norms and the names of tests.
- Quit: Exit the program.

This program is not as user-friendly as those for the AAU test or the FIT-NESSGRAM. It is difficult to correct mistakes, even with the help of the manual. Finally, the software has not been updated since the President's Challenge Test was last revised in 1987.

To purchase this software, contact the following firms:

Harley Courseware, Inc.
3001 Coolidge, Suite 400
East Lansing, MI 48823
800-247-1380
517-333-5325 (fax)

Comptech Software
P.O. Box 107
Waconia, MN 55387
800-343-2406

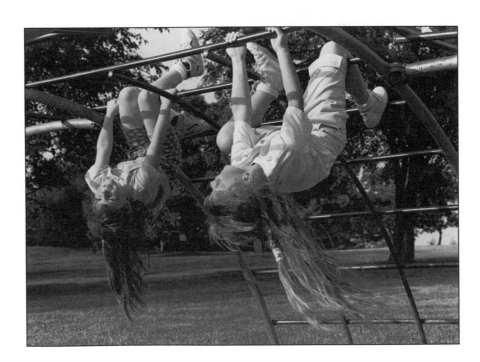

YMCA Youth Fitness Test

Test Sponsor and Developer

YMCA of the USA

Target Population

Ages 6 to 17. No modifications for children with special needs.

Definition of Fitness

Physical fitness is defined as

> one's capacity to achieve the optimal quality of life. It is an ever-changing, many-faceted state that includes healthy mental, social, spiritual, and physical behaviors. . . . The fit person possesses all of the following:
>
> • Cardiorespiratory endurance
> • Mental alertness
> • Meaningful relationships with others
> • Desirable level of fat
> • Desirable level of strength
> • Desirable level of flexibility
> • A healthy low back (Franks, 1989, p. 3)

The YMCA test views five components of fitness as basic:

> • Cardiorespiratory endurance, defined as "the ability of the heart, lungs, and blood vessels to get oxygen to the muscles and the ability of the muscle fibers to use that oxygen to obtain the energy needed for physical activity" (Franks, 1989, p. 6)
> • Relative leanness, defined as "the proportion of fat on the body" (Franks, 1989, p. 7)
> • Healthy low-back function, defined as a low back free of pain
> • Muscular strength and endurance
> • Flexibility, defined as "the ability of a joint to move through a normal range of motion" (Franks, 1989, p. 8)

Tests

Five tests make up the YMCA Youth Fitness Test, shown in Table 3.5.

Two of the tests are notably different versions of tests used in other test batteries. The modified pull-ups test is performed by lifting the body up from the floor until the chest touches an elastic band, then lowering the body and continuing with as many repetitions as possible in correct form up to 20. The curl-ups test is performed with the knees at an angle of 150 degrees and the feet not anchored. The child curls moderately, sliding the hands along the thighs until they reach the knees, then lowers the upper body until the head rests in a partner's hands. There is no time limit, and the child does as many as possible without stopping until up to 40 curl-ups have been performed.

Table 3.5   YMCA Youth Fitness Test Battery

Item	Component of fitness
One-mile run	Cardiorespiratory endurance
Triceps and calf skin-folds	Relative leanness
Sit-and-reach test	Flexibility and healthy low back
Curl-ups	Muscular strength and endurance (abdominals and healthy low back)
Modified pull-ups	Muscular strength and endurance (arms)

Standards and Award System

Criterion-referenced standards are available for this test. There is no award system, other than a certificate for test participation ($4.25 for 10).

Materials

The materials available for this test are a test manual and a youth fitness curriculum manual.

The *YMCA Youth Fitness Test Manual* ($11.50) defines fitness, describes test administration and testing instructions, and briefly discusses applications of test results. It includes the test standards.

The *YMCA Youth Fitness Program* (Thomas, Lee, & Thomas, 1990) curriculum manual ($68) is divided into two parts, one with background information on health-related youth fitness and curriculum use and the other with lesson plans. The lesson plans are further divided into a set for Grades 1 to 3 and set for Grades 4 to 6. Each set contains four 10-week units, with 20 lessons per unit. The lesson format includes presentation of a fitness concept, followed by suggested fitness activities, and then presentation of a health concept. Although the manual was designed for a YMCA setting, it could be equally useful in schools.

These materials are available from the following address:

YMCA Program Store
Box 5076
Champaign, IL 61825-5076
800-747-0089

Software

No software is available.

National Youth Physical Fitness Program

Test Sponsor and Developer

The United States Marines Youth Foundation

Target Population

Ages 5 to 17+. The test has provisions for children with handicaps and those who are underdeveloped or overweight. Modifications of tests and standards are allowed, but not specified. Such modifications are at the discretion of the teacher.

Definition of Fitness

This test identifies four components of physical fitness: upper-body strength, abdominal-muscle strength, leg strength, and agility, speed, and endurance.

Tests

The tests in this test battery appear in Table 3.6.

This test battery differs from those previously described, as it covers fewer health-related components of fitness. Also, although each test is scored separately, the teacher converts the score to a point value and obtains a composite score by adding the point values for the five tests. Composite scores are not usually recommended for fitness test batteries because each test measures a different component of fitness; by creating a composite score, information is lost about the individual components.

Another difference with this test battery is that the developers suggest testing be done in competitive meets; six contestants on each team compete in all events. In the meets, only 3 min are allowed between the administration of each test.

Standards and Award System

The award system consists of a series of 17 Certificates of Athletic Accomplishment. Students earn a certificate each time they attain a score of 250 points or

Table 3.6   National Youth Physical Fitness Program Test Battery

Item	Component of fitness
Sit-ups	Abdominal-muscle strength
Push-ups	Upper-body strength
Modified push-ups	
Standing long jump	Leg strength
Pull-ups	Upper-body strength
Modified pull-ups	
Shuttle run (300 yd)	Agility, speed, and endurance

more. After attaining the first certificate, the student is eligible for the second one the next year, and so on.

Materials

The materials available for the Youth Fitness Program include the following:

- A program booklet
- Award certificates
- A videotape, *The Fitness Challenge*, that depicts the benefits of exercise and good nutrition and displays a series of warm-up exercises demonstrated by the winners of national meets
- A newsletter, *Update: The Fitness Challenge*

The program booklet contains descriptions of the tests, an explanation of the competitive program, sample certificates, and tables of scores with their point equivalents.

The booklet, award certificates, and newsletter are free. The videotape is $29.95 (plus $2.50 shipping and handling). All proceeds from the sale of the videotape benefit the United States Marines Youth Foundation, the nonprofit organization that funds the National Youth Physical Fitness Program.

All materials are available from the following address:

The United States Marines Youth Foundation, Inc.
5700 Monroe St.; P.O. Box 8280
Sylvania, OH 43560
419-882-0051; Ext. 258

Software

No software is available.

Program Comparisons

To help you review the main features of each testing program, we include in this section comparisons of: the tests within each test battery, standards, and available materials and costs.

Tests

The validity of the test battery depends on the objectives of your fitness program. If your objectives are primarily health-related, two batteries focus solely on health-related fitness: FITNESSGRAM and YMCA Youth Fitness Test. If your objectives include some that are performance-related, you might use some of the optional tests from the AAU Test; The President's Challenge and National Youth Fitness Program test batteries are a mixture of health-related and performance-related tests.

Table 3.7 is a summary of the tests included in each battery.

Table 3.7 Tests in Test Batteries

Test battery	Walk/ run	Shuttle runs	Skinfolds	Sit-and-reach	V-sit	Sit-ups	Curl-ups	Pull-ups	Flexed arm hang	Push-ups	Standing long jump	Others
							Tests					
Physical Best	X		X	X		X		X	X	X	X	Body mass index
Chrysler-AAU	X	X		X		X		X	X	X		Hoosier endurance run; phantom chair; sprints
FITNESSGRAM	X	X	X	X			X	X	X			Trunk lift; hip flexor test; body mass index
President's Challenge	X	X		X	X		X	X				
YMCA Youth Fitness	X		X	X			X	X				
National Youth Fitness Program	X	X				X	X	X	X	X		

Table 3.8 provides information on validity, reliability, and objectivity for some of these tests.

One point to keep in mind when you consider which tests to use is that some tests don't reflect good movement principles. For example, in the most widely used version of sit-ups, students' feet are anchored and arms folded across the chest and they are timed for 1 min. This forces the child to hurry in order to execute as many repetitions as possible, yet it is known that a slow curl-up is a better activity for increasing abdominal strength. Another problem occurs with pull-ups. Many children cannot perform even one pull-up, so this test is not a very discriminating measure of upper-body strength and endurance. The modified versions of pull-ups are far more suitable for use in schools than regular pull-ups, because most children can perform the modified ones.

Standards

Criterion-referenced standards are not completely validated at this time. The FITNESSGRAM standards differ from the Physical Best standards, sometimes markedly. For instance, the distance run standard varies between the two tests, in some cases as much as 3 min for a given age and sex. In general the FITNESSGRAM standards are lower (easier) than the Physical Best standards.

In 1990 Cureton and Warren published a study showing that the standards of FITNESSGRAM are more valid than those for Physical Best. In other words, the FITNESSGRAM standards classify students more accurately than the standards for Physical Best. Students who meet the FITNESSGRAM standards also meet minimal health standards and vice versa. AAHPERD has discontinued its use of the Physical Best test and now uses FITNESSGRAM standards. YMCA standards fall between the standards for FITNESSGRAM and Physical Best.

Materials and Cost

All test developers should supply a detailed manual with instructions on administering the test and the program. It should include the following:

- A definition of physical fitness
- Information about the validity and reliability of each item
- Practical tips on administering the test and program

Table 3.8 Validity, Reliability, and Objectivity of Selected Tests

Test	Validity	Reliability*	Objectivity**
One-mile run	Moderate to high	Moderate to high	Moderate to high
Sit-and-reach	Low	High	High
Sit-ups	Moderate	Moderate to high	Moderate
Pull-ups	Moderate	High	Moderate to high
Skinfolds	High	N/A	High

*Assumes adequate motivation of students.
**Assumes sufficient training of testers.

- Samples of appropriate activities for improving performance on the components of fitness included in their fitness definition
- Standards and their basis if they are criterion-referenced

Table 3.9 summarizes the materials available for each testing program and their cost as of the date of publication of this manual. Costs are estimated based on administering the test to 500 children at one time.

The program with the most complete set of materials is FITNESSGRAM. It has videos, curricular materials, a fitness education program, computer software, extensive award systems, a health-related physical fitness test battery, criterion-referenced standards, and a recently-published technical manual. It also has staff available to answer questions on a helpline.

One omission from all test programs is a comprehensive test of fitness knowledge. Both cognitive and affective behaviors have become more important in physical education in recent years, as teachers have emphasized developing lifelong fitness skills. We hope such a test will be added in the near future.

Computer software for physical fitness tests is becoming more user-friendly. Look for a program that doesn't require complicated installation, that displays a menu on the screen as soon as the program is launched, and that can be used

Table 3.9 Comparison of Materials and Costs for Testing Programs

	Chrysler/AAU	FITNESSGRAM	PCPFS	YMCA	Youth Fitness Program
Software	$15	Free	100	None	None
Awards	$10 (shipping)	$52.50 to $437.50	$281.50*	$212.50	Free
Forms	Free	$60**	None	None	Free in booklet
Video	$29.95 $7 (rent)	Available through Prudential agent	None	None	$29.95
Testing manual	Free	Part of special enrollment package ($76)	Free	$11.50	Free
Curriculum manual	3 available, $12 each	$21.95	None	$68	None
Other	Helpline	Helpline	Instructor emblem, $1.50 each	None	None
	Posters: Jungle, $2 each, $7 all four; Motivational, $1 each, $4 all five Special Test Tips, free		Get Fit! booklets, free		

*Assumes an order of 25 Presidential Awards and 250 National Awards.
**Price includes software user's manual.

without frequent reference to a manual. The manual that is included should be written clearly, with attention to detail, no matter how small. Keep in mind that software must be updated continually, which is very expensive, so expect software from programs with corporate backing such as Chrysler Fund/AAU and the Prudential FITNESSGRAM to be revised more frequently than others.

The helpline assistance offered during the work week by Physical Best, FIT-NESSGRAM, and AAU is useful, but not always speedy. We never called without receiving an answer eventually, but we may not have received it on the first, or even second, call. Sometimes the person who could answer the question was out of the office; occasionally, no one would answer the phone at all. Most of the time a staff member responded courteously and helpfully. Because they have larger staffs, FITNESSGRAM and AAU responded more readily. Improvements in helplines would make all packages more attractive.

References

American Alliance for Health, Physical Education, Recreation and Dance (AAHPERD). (1988). *Physical Best*. Reston, VA: Author.

Benham, T.B. (1988). *The A.A.U. developmental physical fitness curricular guide, grades 5-8: Instructor's manual*. Bloomington, IN: Amateur Athletic Union.

Chrysler Fund/Amateur Athletic Union. (1993-94). *Physical Fitness Program*. Bloomington, IN: Author.

Cooper Institute for Aerobics Research. (1992). *The Prudential FITNESSGRAM test administration manual*. Dallas: Author.

Corbin, C.B., & Pangrazi, R.P. (n.d.) *Teaching strategies for improving youth fitness*. Dallas: Cooper Institute for Aerobics Research.

Cureton, K.J., & Warren, G.L. (1990). Criterion-referenced standards for youth health-related fitness: A tutorial. *Research Quarterly for Exercise and Sport*, **61**, 7-19.

Franks, D.B. (1989). *YMCA Youth Fitness Test manual*. Champaign, IL: Human Kinetics.

McSwegin, P., Pemberton, C., Petray, C., & Going, S. (1989). *Physical Best: The AAHPERD guide to physical fitness education and assessment*. Reston, VA: American Alliance for Health, Physical Education, Recreation and Dance.

President's Council on Physical Fitness and Sports. (1993a). *Get fit!: A handbook for youth ages 6-17*. Washington, DC: Author.

President's Council on Physical Fitness and Sports. (1993b). *The President's Challenge Physical Fitness Program packet*. Washington, DC: Author.

Thomas, K.T., Lee, A.M., & Thomas, J.R. (1990). *YMCA Youth Fitness Program*. Champaign, IL: Human Kinetics.

Updyke, W.F. (1987, October). *The trouble with fitness*. Paper presented at the Midwest District Meeting of the American Alliance for Health, Physical Education, Recreation and Dance, Chicago.

CHAPTER 4

Test Descriptions

We've looked at the complete package for each major testing program. Now we'll consider the heart of the matter: the tests in each test battery. For each type of test, we'll answer some questions in these areas:

- *Objective:* What fitness component or components does it measure? Is it more health-related or performance-related?

- *Advantages and disadvantages:* How does this test compare to similar tests? Are there unique problems or advantages to using it?

- *Measurement capabilities:* What is the test's validity and reliability? (These are not always available.)

- *Protocol:* What equipment is needed? What is the starting position? How is the test performed? What's the best way to administer the test?

- *Scoring:* In what units is the scoring done? How are scores to be recorded?

These are the tests we discuss in this chapter, in alphabetical order:

Back saver sit-and-reach   PACER
Body composition   Phantom chair
Curl-ups   Pull-ups
Flexed arm hang   Push-ups
Hoosier endurance shuttle run   Shoulder stretch
Isometric push-ups   Shuttle run
Modified pull-ups   Sit-ups
Modified push-ups   Sit-and-reach test (V-sit and box)
Modified sit-ups   Sprints
90-degree push-ups   Standing long jump
One-mile walk/run   Trunk lift

The test administration instructions in this chapter are generic; they are meant to describe closely similar tests that may appear in various test batteries. Because test procedures often differ from battery to battery, *always review the instructions in the manual published by the test developer before administering any test.*

Back Saver Sit-and-Reach

Objective

Measure hamstring flexibility; health-related

Advantages and Disadvantages

This is a variation on the standard sit-and-reach test that requires the student to place one foot at a time against the sit-and-reach box (see sit-and-reach test). It is recommended by physical therapists who oppose the standard test, which might cause back or hamstring strain: This test is viewed as safer and easier to administer than the standard test. It measures only hamstring flexibility, however, not lower back flexibility.

Protocol

Equipment: This test requires a standard sit-and-reach box (or any box roughly 12 in. high), with the measuring stick positioned on top of the box so that the 9-in. mark is on the near edge of the box.

Starting position: After removing shoes, the student sits with one leg straight out, the foot flat against the front of the box, and the other leg bent with the foot flat on the floor about 2 in. to 3 in. from the inside of the opposite leg. Hips should be parallel to the box. The zero point on the measuring stick is closest to the student.

Performance: The student places one hand on top of the other, palms down, and reaches as far as possible four times, moving the hands across the top of the box. On the fourth try, the position is held for at least a second. The same should be done with the opposite leg.

Scoring

Two scores are recorded, one for each side. The score is recorded in inches to the last whole inch reached, with a maximum score of 12. Results are classified as either pass or fail.

Body Composition: Skinfold Measurements or Body Mass Index

Objective

Measure body composition; health-related

Advantages and Disadvantages

Of the two forms of body composition measurement, skinfold measurement is more accurate: The body mass index does not distinguish body fat from lean body mass. However, skinfold measurement requires more time than simply taking a student's height and weight.

One disadvantage of skinfold measurement is that test reliability depends on the skill of the tester. It's important that testers practice a lot before working in a real test situation.

Students should learn that it is possible to weigh too little, as well as too much. In the Prudential FITNESSGRAM program, the score is flagged with a special message if the percent fat is above or below a certain standard. For boys 12 and older the low-fat message prints at 8% body fat; for girls of the same age, it prints at 13% body fat. The message about being too thin does not print for children under 12.

Measurement Capabilities

Validity: For skinfold measurements, the validity is .70 to .90 when compared with body fatness measured by hydrostatic weighing.

Reliability: For skinfold measurements, reliability is greater than .95 between testers.

Protocol

Equipment: A skinfold caliper is required to take skinfold measurements. For body mass index, a measuring stick and a scale are needed to measure height and weight.

Performance: In general, skinfold thickness measures are taken at the triceps and the calf, always (for consistency) on the right side of the body.

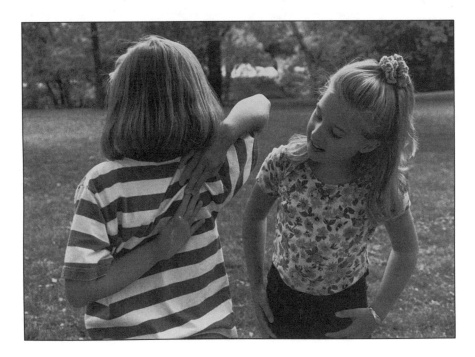

(FITNESSGRAM also offers standards for abdominal site measurements for college-age students only.) The test instructions typically describe a precise method for locating the skinfold site. By pinching the fold slightly above the midpoint of the site, the tester can place the caliper at the midpoint. The tester holds the caliper in position for 3 sec and records the measurement. Each site is measured three times.

Some testers feel the calf site is a bit more difficult to measure than the triceps site. It helps to have the student position the knee at a 90-degree angle and try to relax the calf. Testers should practice measuring skinfolds many times before testing students and should follow test directions carefully. For body mass calculations, testers should measure students' height and weight.

Scoring

Skinfold thickness is measured in millimeters, the scale on the dial of the caliper. Each skinfold is measured three times, but the highest and lowest measurements are discarded. Only the middle score of the three is recorded.

The following formula determines body mass:

$$\text{Weight(kg)}/\text{height(m)}^2$$

Fitness test computer software usually calculates this value automatically when given weight in pounds and height in inches. If it doesn't, record weight and height in kilograms and meters.

Curl-Ups

Objective

Measure strength and endurance of abdominal muscles; health-related

Advantages and Disadvantages

This test is a good alternative to sit-ups. First, sit-ups require the child to come up to a sitting position. This means that during the last half of the sit-up the child is primarily using hip flexors instead of abdominal muscles. Curl-ups raise the upper back off the mat in a curled position, which eliminates the use of the hip flexors. In addition, students perform curl-ups to a cadence, instead of being timed. Timed tests may result in incorrect form because a child may hurry in order to do as many sit-ups as possible. Finally, differences in body proportion between children affect curl-up performance very little. Overall curl-ups are mechanically more appropriate and thus more valid than either sit-ups or modified sit-ups.

Protocol

Equipment: This test requires a floor mat; in the Prudential FITNESSGRAM test, a cardboard measuring strip is recommended. The strip should be 30 in. × 4-1/2 in. for 10- to 17-year-olds and 30 in. × 3 in. for 5- to 9-year-olds.

Starting position: The FITNESSGRAM version groups students by threes. As one student takes the test, another stands with both feet on the ends of the measuring strip. The third student places both hands under the head of the student being tested and counts the repetitions. Partners must be properly trained so they do not obstruct testing.

The YMCA version pairs the students. The assisting student places both hands under the head of the student being tested.

The student being tested lies on the mat, with knees bent and feet flat on the floor. In the FITNESSGRAM version, arms and hands are held straight at the sides, with palms in contact with the mat. Fingertips touch the near edge of the measuring strip. In the YMCA version the hands rest on the thighs. For both versions the head is in a partner's hands on the floor.

Performance: In the FITNESSGRAM version, the student curls up until the fingertips touch the far edge of the strip, then lowers the upper body until the head touches the hands on the mat. Repetitions are performed to a cadence of one curl-up every 3 sec (The cadence can be provided by playing an audiocassette tape, clapping hands, or beating a drum.)

In the YMCA version, the student curls up until the fingertips touch the knees. One curl-up is to be done about every 3 sec, but there is no cadence.

For the FITNESSGRAM version the student continues performing curl-ups until no more can be performed or 75 have been completed. For the YMCA version, the student stops when he or she quits or performs 40, is unable to maintain correct rhythm after three tries, has made three errors in technique, or experiences discomfort or pain.

Scoring

The score is the number of curl-ups performed with correct form. Heels must stay on the mat during the curl, and the student must curl from the spine up. A curl is counted when the student's head touches the assisting student's hands.

Flexed Arm Hang

Objective

Measure upper-body arm as well as shoulder girdle strength and endurance; health-related

Advantages and Disadvantages

This test is an alternative to pull-ups that can be used for just girls or boys and girls. The advantage of this test over pull-ups is that most children can perform this test, whereas many cannot perform pull-ups at all. The disadvantage is that this test is difficult to administer—some children must be lifted to the bar and timing is sometimes imprecise—and it requires one-on-one testing.

Performance on pull-ups and flexed arm hang is negatively correlated with weight, presumably because of the inverse relationship between the number of pull-ups performed and body fatness. These two tests do correlate moderately with each other.

Measurement Capabilities

Validity: The validity is .72 when compared to pull-ups.

Reliability: The reliability is .74 to .89.

Protocol

Equipment: This test requires a chinning bar, a mat, and a stopwatch.

Starting position: The student grabs the bar using the grip designated in the test instructions. The tester may assist the student in lifting the body until the chin is above the bar.

Performance: The tester starts the stopwatch as soon as the student is in the starting position. The student holds the position as long as he or she can, not allowing the body to swing. As soon as the student can no longer hold the chin above the bar the tester stops timing.

Scoring

The score is the length of time the correct position is held. It is recorded in seconds and, in the AAU version, tenths of seconds.

Hoosier Endurance Shuttle Run

Objective

Measure cardiorespiratory endurance (aerobic capacity); health-related

Advantages and Disadvantages

This is a new modification of the 20-m shuttle test (see PACER described later). Presently no information is available on how this test compares with other shuttle runs or the one-mile walk/run. It would be expected to have a low to moderate correlation with shuttle run tests other than the 20-m shuttle run, because those tests are designed primarily to measure agility rather than aerobic capacity. It should have a relatively high correlation with the one-mile walk/run or the 20-m shuttle run, which are valid measures of aerobic capacity.

According to the test developer, this test is fun and motivating for students. It also can be administered indoors with groups of students. However, setting up this test is more work than setting up comparable tests. Also, the speed of the run does not increase during the test, as it does in the 20-m shuttle run, and the fact that the student must pick up and drop a ball introduces an element of performance other than aerobic capacity into the test. This test may turn out to be more of a measure of agility and speed than aerobic capacity.

Protocol

Equipment: Each child must have 15 tennis balls, two chairs (or traffic cones), and one box for collecting the balls. The test administrator needs a stopwatch and a large ball-supply box. Draw lines in front of each line of chairs (or cones), which are 20 yd apart.

Starting position: Pair students. The student being tested stands with a foot touching the line by the first chair. The partner stands behind the second chair with the tennis balls and places a ball on that chair.

Performance: The student runs to the second chair and picks up the ball, returns to the first chair (chair seat facing away from the runner), runs around it, and drops the ball in a box on the seat of that chair. As soon as the participant picks up the first ball the partner places another ball on the second chair. The object of the test is to collect as many balls as possible in a given time period, 6 min for 6- to 11-year-olds and 9 min for 12- to 17-year-olds. Students may walk.

Scoring

The score is the number of balls picked up during the test.

Isometric Push-Ups

Objective

Measure upper-body muscular strength and endurance; health-related

Advantages and Disadvantages

This is another alternative to push-ups. Most students can score on this test, and it has the added advantage that it can be administered to a large group of students at one time. But it is difficult to monitor the 90-degree angle at the elbow because there's no way to judge how much the angle may change before the test is stopped.

This test is limited by the fact that it only measures isometric strength and endurance. It also may be an easier test for shorter, more muscular students than for taller, leaner students.

Protocol

Equipment: This test requires a mat and a stopwatch.

Starting position: The student lies prone on the mat, hands on the mat next to the chest and elbows bent.

Performance: On a signal, the student pushes the body up until his or her elbows reach an angle of 90 degrees, holding this position as long as possible.

Scoring

The score is the time the position is held to nearest tenth of a second.

Modified Pull-Ups

Objective

Measure upper-body muscular strength and endurance; health-related

Advantages and Disadvantages

This test is a good alternative to pull-ups, as more children are able to perform this test than pull-ups. However, it is difficult to ensure that students maintain correct form throughout the test so testing must be done one-on-one. It also requires special equipment, but that equipment can be built easily.

Measurement Capabilities

(For modified pull-ups with stand)

Validity: The validity is satisfactory when compared with tests of arm and shoulder girdle strength using a weight training machine.

Reliability: Reliability is .71 for elementary school, .98 for high school.

Protocol

Equipment: You will need a modified pull-up stand (instructions for building this stand appear in Appendix B.) for the FITNESSGRAM and YMCA versions (see Figure 4.1); a horizontal bar that can be adjusted in height for the National Youth Physical Fitness Program (NYPFP) version.

Starting position: For the FITNESSGRAM and YMCA versions, the student assumes a hanging position with an overhand grip (palms away from the body), arms straight, body straight, and heels touching the floor. The bar is adjusted so it is 1 in. to 2 in. above the child's grasp while lying on the floor, so that the body is not touching the mat. An elastic band is positioned 7 in. to 8 in. below the bar.

For the NYPFP version, students are paired. The student being tested grabs the bar with an overhand grip, keeping the head, trunk, and legs in a straight line and heels on the floor. The arms are straightened at a 90-degree angle to the trunk. The partner holds the student's heels to keep the feet stable.

Performance: In the FITNESSGRAM and YMCA versions, the student pulls up on a signal until the elastic band touches just below the chin. The student then lowers the body to the straight arm position and continues performing modified pull-ups without stopping.

A partner can help check that the student performs repetitions with correct form. Each time the body is lowered, the arms must be straightened completely. If the student bends at the hips or knees, the pull-up doesn't count. The body

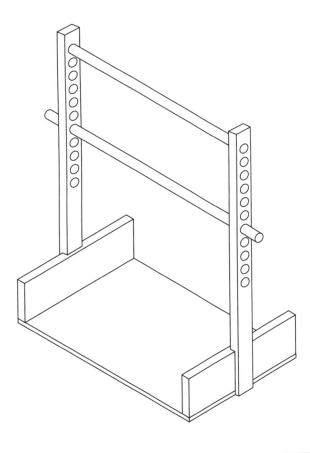

Figure 4.1   A modified pull-up stand.
Adapted with permission from Cooper Institute for Aerobics Research, Dallas, TX.

should be held as a rigid bar. If the body moves up and down, in a wave, the pull-up doesn't count.

In the YMCA version, the test is stopped after the student performs three incorrect pull-ups, completes 20 correctly, or complains of low-back pain. In the FITNESSGRAM version, the test is stopped if the student experiences extreme discomfort or pain.

In the NYPFP version, the student pulls the chest up to the bar. He or she then extends the arms back to the starting position. This motion is repeated continuously for 2 min.

Scoring

The score is the total number of pull-ups performed correctly. In the NYPFP version, points are given on the basis of the number of pull-ups.

Modified Push-Ups

Objective

Measure upper-body muscular strength and endurance; health-related

Advantages and Disadvantages

This is a slightly easier version of the push-up, which means that students are more likely to be able to do at least one. It also can be administered to a large group of students at the same time.

Monitoring both the alignment of the body and the angle at the elbow can be difficult. As no cadence is used, it's also possible that some students may perform the modified push-ups too rapidly and with poor form.

Protocol

Equipment: This test requires a mat and a stopwatch.

Starting position: For the AAU version, the student lies prone on the mat, hands next to the chest and elbows bent. The lower legs are crossed with knees bent. For the NYPFP version, the student begins with arms straight, hands on the mat under and a bit outside of the shoulders, and knees bent at a 90-degree angle to the thighs. The rest of the body is held straight. A partner lies on the mat facing the student and places a hand under the student's chest.

Performance: In the AAU version, the student pushes up on a signal raising the body until the arms are straight. Body weight should be balanced on the hands and knees, and the body should be held in a straight line. The student then bends the arms and lowers the chest to the mat to complete one push-up, doing as many of these as possible in 30 sec.

In the NYPFP version, the student keeps the body straight, lowers the chest until it touches the partner's hand, and then straightens the arms to return to the starting position. The student does as many of these as possible in 2 min.

Scoring

The score is the number of push-ups done correctly within the time period. The NYPFP version gives points based on the number of push-ups.

Modified Sit-Ups

This test is essentially the same as sit-ups (described later) with arms crossed over the chest, except that the student is required to curl up until the *elbows*, rather than the forearms, touch the thighs and to curl down to only about the shoulders. (The curl-up in the President's Challenge Test is a modified sit-up.)

90-Degree Push-Ups

Objective

Measure upper-body muscular strength and endurance; health-related

Advantages and Disadvantages

This test is another alternative to pull-ups. Again, most children can perform at least one repetition of the 90-degree push-ups, which has the advantage over pull-ups and modified pull-ups in that it can be administered to a group of students instead of one-on-one. It is difficult, however, for students to maintain proper form throughout the test and for someone to monitor the students' performance.

Protocol

Equipment: This test requires a floor mat, a tape with a 20 beat per minute cadence, and a cassette player.

Starting position: Students work in pairs so one can monitor the position of the other during test performance. The student performing the exercise lies face down on the mat in standard push-up position: hands under shoulders, fingers straight, and legs straight, parallel, and slightly apart, with the toes supporting the feet.

Performance: The student straightens the arms, keeping the back and knees straight, then lowers the arms until there is a 90-degree angle at the elbows (upper arms will be parallel to the floor). The partner, kneeling in front of the participant, counts and watches to see that the angle of the elbow is 90 degrees each time a push-up is performed.

The student performs as many push-ups as possible, maintaining a cadence of 20 per min. The test is over when the student can no longer perform the push-up with the correct positioning (three corrections are allowed), is in pain, or stops.

Scoring

The score is the number of repetitions performed correctly. Incorrect performance occurs when the participant cannot perform at the designated cadence or the form is incorrect (knees bent to the mat, back swayed, incomplete arm extension, jerky movement, no 90-degree angle at the elbow).

One-Mile Walk/Run

Objective

Measure cardiorespiratory endurance; health-related

Advantages and Disadvantages

This is a valid, easy-to-use test of aerobic capacity that is accurate when students perform at their maximum. However, it must be administered outdoors, and it is sometimes hard to motivate students to give their full effort during the test.

Some test batteries require children of all ages to take this test. Shorter distances are recommended for younger children in the AAU test: 1/4 mi. for

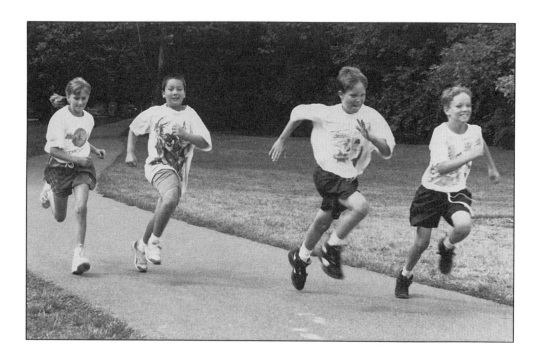

6- to 7-year-olds, 1/2 mi. for 8- to 9-year-olds, and 3/4 mi. for 10- to 11-year-olds. The PACER is recommended instead for children in Grades K to 3 by FITNESSGRAM. The validity of shorter distances is somewhat lower, but it is often difficult to motivate younger children to run a whole mile.

Measurement Capabilities

Validity: Validity is .71 to .81 when compared with maximum oxygen uptake measured from a maximum stress test.

Reliability: Reliability coefficients range from .40 to .98.

Protocol

Equipment: You will need a measured running area (including a line marker) and a stopwatch.

Starting positions: Students line up behind the starting line. Remind them to use a controlled pace so they can finish the run.

Performance: On a signal students begin running. Walking is allowed, although students are encouraged to finish the course as quickly as possible. Record times as each student crosses the finish line. Use a partner as the scorer for each child to facilitate scoring.

Scoring

The time taken to complete the run is recorded in minutes and seconds. In the Prudential FITNESSGRAM test the computer program transforms the time to a $\dot{V}O_2$max reading, and this is also reported on the FITNESSGRAM report card.

PACER

Objective

Measure cardiorespiratory endurance; health-related

Advantages and Disadvantages

This is a valid test that is highly motivating to students and can be administered indoors. Its only disadvantage is that it may take students some time to learn.

Measurement Capabilities

Validity: Validity is .52 to .93 when compared with maximum oxygen uptake measured from a maximum stress test on the treadmill.

Reliability: Reliability coefficients range from .89 to .98.

Protocol

Equipment: This test requires a cassette tape player, an audiocassette tape with timed "beeps" recorded, marker cones, pencils, and scoring sheets. (The Prudential FITNESSGRAM program provides a tape with the beeps, along with a version with music in the background, if desired.) Lines are placed on the floor 20 m (21 yd and 32 in.) apart.

Starting position: The students line up behind one line. Each student should have a partner to record laps.

Performance: The tape starts with a countdown of 5-4-3-2-1 followed by the command "Begin." On this command students begin running toward the other line. The run should be paced so that they reach the other line at the first beep (9 sec). (The speed begins at 8.5 km/h-1 and increases 0.5 km/h-1 at each successive minute. When three beeps are heard at the end of a lap, the distance from one line to another, the speed increases.) Students touch the line, turn around, and run toward the starting line, again timing the run to reach the line at the sound of the next beep. They continue running back and forth until they can no longer keep up the pace. When someone misses reaching the lines for three beeps the test stops for that student.

For students in Grades K to 3, this test is used more as a fun activity. Students are allowed to run as long as they like (usually not more than a few minutes).

Scoring

A point is scored for each completed lap. The Prudential FITNESSGRAM software automatically converts this score to a $\dot{V}O_2$max reading.

For children in Grades K to 3, a score of "0" laps is entered to indicate they finished the test.

Phantom Chair

Objective

Measure static-leg endurance; performance-related

Advantages and Disadvantages

This test of leg muscle endurance is easy to administer, but it has not been assessed for validity. It would seem to have logical validity, as leg strength is clearly required to perform the test.

Protocol

Equipment: You will need a stopwatch and an exercise mat.

Starting position: The student stands with the back against a wall and feet flat on a mat.

Performance: The student slides down the wall until the knees reach a 90-degree angle, with the arms hanging at the sides. This forms a mock sitting position with the body. The feet should be flat and pointed forward. The student holds this position as long as possible.

Scoring

The score is the time from the moment the correct position is assumed until this position can no longer be maintained. The time is recorded to the nearest second.

Pull-Ups

Objective

Measure upper-body strength and endurance; health-related

Advantages and Disadvantages

Most instructors and students are familiar with this test. As many students cannot perform even one repetition of this test, though, test developers are beginning to use alternative tests such as the flexed arm hang or push-ups. This test also requires one-on-one testing. Pull-ups performance is negatively correlated with body weight.

Measurement Capabilities

Validity: The validity of this test is logical.

Reliability: The reliability of this test is .89.

Protocol

Equipment: For pull-ups you need a horizontal bar secured at a height at which all students can hang from the bar without their feet touching the floor.

Starting position: The student grasps the bar and hangs with arms and body straight. The tester is permitted to assist the student in reaching the bar in the FITNESSGRAM and President's Challenge versions. Most tests require an overhand grip with palms facing away from the body, although the AAU test now allows children to choose either an overhand or underhand grip.

Performance: The student uses the arms to lift the body up until the chin is above the bar, then lowers the body to the hanging position. The student performs as many pull-ups as possible without bending or kicking the legs or swinging the body.

Scoring

The score is the number of correctly completed pull-ups. The FITNESSGRAM computer program does not accept a zero score for pull-ups, so if a student cannot perform at least one pull-up, another test that measures upper-body strength and endurance must be selected. In the NYPFP version, points are given for the number of pull-ups.

Push-Ups

Objective

Measure upper-body muscular strength and endurance; health-related

Advantages and Disadvantages

Most children are familiar with this test, and it can be administered to a large group of students at the same time. Its largest disadvantage is that many children cannot perform even one push-up, so it cannot be used as a measurement for them. Maintaining good form throughout the push-up is difficult, and judging acceptable from unacceptable form in order to score also is difficult.

Measurement Capabilities

Validity: The validity is logical.

Reliability: The reliability is .83 to .97.

Protocol

Equipment: You will need a floor mat.

Starting position: Students work in pairs so one can count repetitions. The student counting lies face down on the mat opposite the student being tested and places his or her hand palm down underneath the tested student. The student performing the exercise has hands on the mat underneath the shoulders, elbows locked. The body is straight, with no part other than the hands and toes touching the mat. Feet are 12 in. or less apart.

Performance: Students bend their arms, lowering the body until the chest touches the counting student's hand and pushing back up to the beginning position. The body must remain straight throughout the movement. Students perform as many push-ups as possible without stopping.

Scoring

The score is the points given based on the number of repetitions performed correctly (this test is part of the NYPFP battery).

Shoulder Stretch

Objective

Measure arm and shoulder flexibility; health-related

Advantages and Disadvantages

This is a simple test that is easy to administer, but it is only a rough measure of arm and shoulder flexibility.

Protocol

Equipment: None

Starting position: Students are paired off so one can watch and judge the completeness of the stretch. The student being tested stands.

Performance: Students first reach their right hand over their right shoulder and down the back. They then bring their left hand underneath their left shoulder and up the back, attempting to reach the fingertips of their right hand.

Students return to normal standing position, repeating the same movements with their left hand reaching over their left shoulder and their right hand reaching underneath their right shoulder.

Scoring

Two scores are recorded, one for the right shoulder and one for the left. A score of Pass is given if the fingertips touch; if they don't, a score of Fail is given.

Shuttle Run

Objective

Measure agility; performance-related

Advantages and Disadvantages

This is a fun test for students, although its validity is questionable. It should not relate highly to the 20-m shuttle run, the PACER, or distance run tests because it is not a measure of aerobic capacity.

Measurement Capabilities

(for the President's Challenge and AAU versions)

Validity: The validity is logical (but questionable).

Reliability: Reliability coefficients range from .68 to .75.

Protocol

Equipment: In the President's Challenge and AAU versions each student needs two (or three) blocks of wood (approximately 2 in. × 2 in. × 4 in.) or two (or three) blackboard erasers, with a stopwatch available, and two lines marked on the floor, 30 ft apart. The NYPFP version requires two markers spaced 60 yd apart, a stopwatch, and a starting pistol.

Starting position: The student stands behind the starting line. In the President's Challenge version, the two blocks of wood or erasers are placed on the floor just beyond the far line. In the AAU version, two blocks are placed just on the far line and one on the starting line.

For the NYPFP version, the student begins in a standing (distance) or crouched (sprinter's) start position. Starting blocks or depressions are not allowed, and the student's entire body must be behind the starting line.

Performance: In the President's Challenge version, students start on a signal, run to the far line, pick up one of the blocks or erasers, return to the starting line, and place the item on the floor beyond the line. They then run back to the far line, pick up the second item, and return to cross the starting line.

In the AAU version, students start on a signal, run to the far line, pick up one of the blocks or erasers, run back to the starting line, and place the item down. They then pick up a second item and run back to the far line, placing the item on the line, picking up the third item, and running as fast as possible back to the starting line.

In the NYPFP version, the student runs the marked distance five times, going completely around each marker.

Scoring

The score is the time from the signal to the instant the student crosses the starting line with the last block or eraser in hand, recorded to the nearest tenth of a second. The blocks or erasers must be placed on the floor, not thrown. For the NYPFP version, the score is a number of points based on the time elapsed, in minutes and seconds, when the student goes past the last marker. If the student doesn't finish the run, no points are awarded.

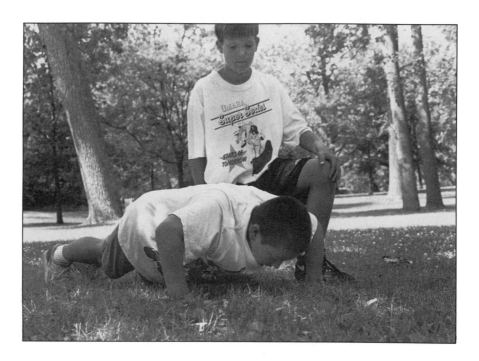

Sit-Ups

Objective

Measure strength and endurance of abdominal muscle; health-related

Advantages and Disadvantages

This test is popular because it can be administered to groups and students are usually familiar with it. But coming up to a full sitting position is unnecessary to measure abdominal strength; the latter part of the sit-up primarily uses the hip flexors. Performing as many sit-ups as possible in a minute also encourages students to use improper form, which can lead to injuries. In addition, body proportions are more likely to affect the results of this test than of curl-ups. If a person has long legs and a short trunk, the sit-up is easier; if a person has short legs and a long trunk, it is harder.

Measurement Capabilities

Validity: The validity is logical.

Reliability: Reliability is .68 to .94.

Protocol

Equipment: This test requires an exercise mat and a stopwatch.

Starting position: Students are paired. The student being tested lies on the back with knees bent and feet flat on the floor. In the AAU version students cross arms on the chest; in the NYPFP they clasp hands behind their head. The partner holds the ankles or feet.

Performance: On a signal the student curls up to a designated point. In the AAU version the forearms (not the elbows) must touch the thighs. In the NYPFP the forehead comes above or in front of the knees. The student then curls the body down to the starting position. For the NYPFP the backs of the hands must touch the mat. The student performs as many sit-ups as possible in 1 (AAU) or 2 (NYPFP) min. Students are allowed to rest.

Scoring

For the AAU version, the score is the number of sit-ups correctly performed during the time limit. For the NYPFP, points are given based on the number of sit-ups.

Sit-and-Reach Test

Two versions of this text exist: One uses a V-sit position, the other uses a sit-and-reach box. Both are described here.

V-Sit

Objective

Measure hamstring flexibility; health-related

Advantages and Disadvantages

The V-sit version of the sit-and-reach test does not require the equipment that the box version does, but it hyperextends the back more. Like the box version, it requires one-on-one testing.

Protocol

Equipment: The V-sit test requires a tape measure or yardstick, which is taped to the floor.

Starting position: Students are paired. The student being tested sits on the floor and straddles the tape or yardstick with the heels 8 in. to 12 in. apart. The heels are lined up along a set mark on the tape or yardstick. The partner holds down the student's ankles for stability or knees to keep them flat.

Performance: Keeping the legs straight, the student slides the hands, palms down, along the tape or yardstick as far as possible. The student repeats the reach for three or four trials.

Scoring

The score is either the farthest distance reached in three trials or the fourth trial. The score should be recorded to either the nearest inch or half-inch, depending on the test protocol.

Box Version

Objective

Measure hamstring flexibility; health-related

Advantages and Disadvantages

This test is easy to administer and is a valid measure of hamstring flexibility. It does not require as much hyperextension of the back as the V-sit version. It does, however, require special equipment and one-on-one testing. It also does not measure lower back flexibility well and is viewed by some physical therapists as an unsafe stretch.

Measurement Capabilities

Validity: The box version validity is .60 to .73 compared with hamstring flexor strength and .27 to .30 compared with lower back flexor strength.

Reliability: Reliability is .70 or higher.

Protocol

Equipment: The box version requires a sit-and-reach box with a measuring scale on top of the box (Instructions on building one appear in Appendix B).

Starting position: The student sits on the floor with feet placed against the sit-and-reach box, legs straight out.

Performance: With legs straight, the student stretches forward along the top of the box four times, hands on top of each other and palms down. On the fourth stretch, he or she reaches as far as possible and holds it for at least a second.

Scoring

The score is the farthest point reached on the fourth stretch to the nearest centimeter or half-inch (depending on the measuring scale on the box).

Sprints

Objective

Measure speed; performance-related

Advantages and Disadvantages

This test is easy to administer and is motivating to many children. But if students are not trained to use an efficient running style, the test is more likely to measure skill in running than an aspect of performance-related physical fitness. Because this test usually must be administered outdoors, test administration is dependent on the weather.

Measurement Capabilities

Validity: The test's validity is logical, but measures running efficiency as well as pure speed.

Reliability: For the 50-yd dash, reliability ranges from .83 to .95.

Protocol

Equipment: This test requires a measured course and a stopwatch. For the AAU version, course length is 50 yd for children 6 to 12 and 100 yd for children 13 to 17.

Starting position: Students stand behind the starting line. Any position is acceptable.

Performance: On a signal, the students run the course as fast as possible.

Scoring

The time taken to run the course is measured to the nearest tenth of a second.

Standing Long Jump

Objective

Measure explosive power of the legs; performance-related

Advantages and Disadvantages

This familiar test is easy to administer, although it requires one-on-one testing.

Protocol

Equipment: You will need a tape measure, a marked line, and a soft area such as a mat or sand pit.

Starting position: The student stands behind the line with feet apart. He or she bends the knees and swings the arms back and forth to prepare for the jump.

Performance: The student jumps forward, landing on one or both feet; three jumps are taken.

Scoring

The score is the distance (in feet and inches) that the student jumps from the line to the point where the heel closest to the line lands. The NYPFP version gives points based on the distance.

Only the best of the three jumps is recorded. (In the NYPFP version, if the student steps over the line, the jump is a foul.) If the student falls or steps backward after landing, the measurement is taken from whatever part of the body touches down closest to the line, rather than the original landing spot.

Trunk Lift (Extension)

Objective

Measure trunk extensor flexibility; health-related

Advantages and Disadvantages

This test requires little equipment and is easy to administer. It does, however, require one-on-one testing, and may lead to overarching the back.

Protocol

Equipment: A foot-long ruler, marked with colored tape at the 6- and 12-in. marks, and a floor mat.

Starting position: The student being tested lies face down, with the hands under the thighs and toes pointed.

Performance: The student lifts the head and upper body and holds that position briefly so it can be measured. (The student should not be encouraged to lift higher than the 12 in. ruler.) The tester measures the distance from the floor to the chin with the ruler. The participant then lowers the upper body down. Two trials are made, with the highest score recorded.

Scoring

The score is the height to which the student was able to lift the upper body, measured from the chin to the floor, recorded to the nearest inch. If the lift exceeds 12 in., it is recorded as 12 in.

References

Jackson, A.W., & Baker, A.A. (1986). The relationship of the Sit-and-Reach Test to criterion measures of hamstring and back flexibility in young females. *Research Quarterly for Exercise and Sport,* **57,** 183-186.

Lohman, T.J. (1987). The use of skinfolds to estimate body fatness of children and youth. *Journal of Physical Education, Recreation and Dance,* **58,** 98-102.

CHAPTER 5

Developing Your Own Test Battery

What if none of the available test batteries suit your needs—should you consider developing one of your own? It's not impossible to do, but it takes a lot of careful planning and hard work. You might first consider those test batteries such as the AAU Test and the Prudential FITNESSGRAM that offer you several options for particular fitness components. Then, if you find that these don't give you the flexibility you desire, you might consider developing a test battery.

The advantages of creating your own test battery include

- choosing the components of fitness you think are most important,
- tailoring your tests to your facilities or students, and
- developing local standards.

You will also face the disadvantages of

- the lack of ready-to-use computer programs, curricular materials, or testing materials (such as scoring cards) available with national test batteries;
- the need to revise your battery yourself on a continuous basis;
- the need to create your own norms and standards; and
- the need to develop your own award system and awards.

If the advantages outweigh the disadvantages for you, then take these steps to develop your test battery:

1. Determine the important components of fitness.
2. Select a test for each component.
3. Try the test battery on a small group.
4. Revise the test battery.
5. Administer the revised test battery to the total group.
6. Develop local norms and standards.
7. Continue to revise your test battery.
8. Develop your own curricular materials.
9. Develop your own award system.

Let's cover each step in more detail.

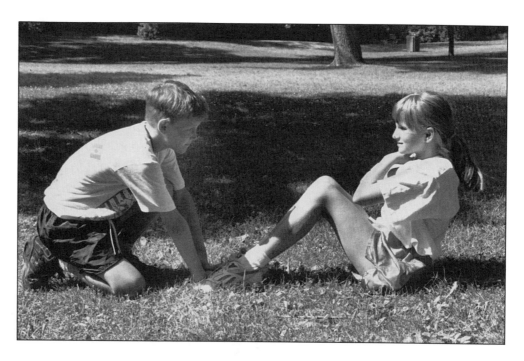

Determine the Important Components of Fitness

How do you define *physical fitness*? The current test batteries typically identify four components of fitness: cardiorespiratory endurance, body composition, muscular strength and endurance, and flexibility. You may wish to add other components, such as balance. Or you may want to cover the same components, but prefer to measure them for different parts of the body. For example, muscular strength and endurance typically is measured for the upper body or abdominals. You may feel it's important to measure strength in other parts of the body, such as the trunk or legs. Another example is flexibility. Tests often measure hamstring flexibility; but since flexibility is specific to each part of the body, you may prefer to test the trunk or shoulders.

Another possibility is including tests with health-related and performance-related elements in your test battery. Speed is a good example. Although health-related fitness is a factor in being able to run fast, this ability primarily reflects performance-related ability. Agility is another performance-related element you might want to include.

Once you've decided on the components of fitness you wish to measure, make sure you can defend the total package as a reflection of your definition of physical fitness. Children frequently ask, "Why do we have to take this test?" You need to be able to explain what each test measures and why that component is important.

Select a Test for Each Component

Once you have identified your components of fitness, select a test to measure each one. Most of the tests in national test batteries have acceptable validity, so you may want to pick and choose your tests from them. If trunk strength is one of your components, the trunk lift test from the FITNESSGRAM test might be an option. Some of the shuttle runs from national batteries measure agility.

You also have the option of designing your own test. A leg press using a weight machine could measure leg strength. Running a short distance, such as 50 yd, could measure speed. Establish your test's validity and reliability, however, before you use it. Administering an invalid test is a waste of time for you and your students. Don't let this discourage you from trying to develop a test, though; a novel test might be a lot more fun for your students than a standard one.

Try the Test Battery on a Small Group

Before you use the battery of tests you've developed on a full-scale basis, administer it to a small group. This lets you find out if there are problems. Do any of the tests take too much time? Can most students obtain a score on all of the tests? Tests that many children cannot perform, such as pull-ups, provide no information about those children's fitness levels.

Before administering your trial version to a few students, properly prepare them to take these tests. Just as with standard tests, students must learn how to perform each test if they are to concentrate on doing their best during testing. If a distance run is part of your test battery, make sure students have practiced running this distance regularly for several weeks prior to testing.

Revise the Test Battery

Once you have administered the test battery on a trial basis, revise the tests based on your observations of problems before, during, and after testing. Was your preparation for testing adequate? Were there problems in administering the test (such as students having trouble following directions)? Ask students for their suggestions. Develop ideas on how to eliminate the problems that occurred. Amend and record testing procedures and file them for future use.

Keeping written records of the problems and possible solutions helps in future test administration. Often we learn a lot about how to improve testing procedures when we administer a test battery, but then forget what we've learned by the next time. Write down what you've learned, listing the potential problems, and review those notes each time you test.

Remember that administering a test battery to a small group does not take as much time as to a large group. If any of the tests you selected or developed are too time-consuming or difficult to use with large numbers of children, drop them and choose or create others. Be sure that the replacement test measures the same component as the original, or the validity of the test battery will be reduced.

Administer the Revised Test Battery to the Total Group

Prepare to administer the revised test battery by creating appropriate score cards or sheets and planning how you will organize testing. You may want to

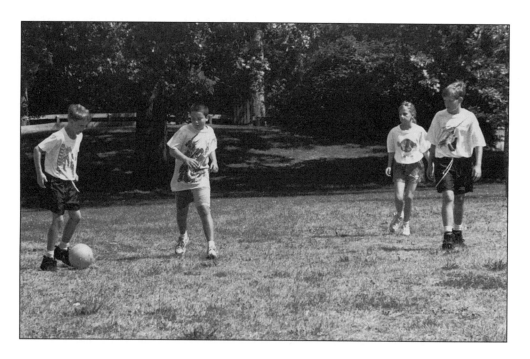

use testing stations, where students rotate from test to test (see "Test Scheduling and Site Organization" in chapter 6). If so, teach students how to use this system prior to testing. Be sure that all students practice each test before you administer the test battery.

Be sure to record scores from testing in order to develop local norms and standards. One of the disadvantages of developing your own test battery is that no norms or standards are available. If your test battery includes tests from various national test batteries, don't compare results across tests. Each set of test standards was determined on a different premise, so they are not comparable.

Develop Local Norms and Standards

Developing local norms requires collecting a substantial set of scores, preferably several hundred for each age group and sex. If this size group is not readily available, accumulate test scores over several test periods. Once enough scores are gathered, a table of percentiles can be developed. We advise that this only be done by computer, not by hand. Once this table is complete, any percentile can be chosen as a standard. For example, the President's Council uses the 85th percentile for the Presidential Physical Fitness Award and the 50th percentile for the National Physical Fitness Award.

Although health-related standards are typically more desirable, they are considerably more difficult to determine. The scores selected as standards must be directly tied to children's health. Even the most experienced fitness test developers have had problems accomplishing this task. Health-related standards for cardiorespiratory endurance and body composition have a relatively sound foundation, but other standards have been determined somewhat arbitrarily. Even those, though, were chosen only after a thorough review of the literature and consideration of the performance levels of children. If you want to use health-related standards, your best choice is to find a test from a national test battery that is very close to yours and use the standards from that test. Otherwise you will have to arbitrarily set standards that will be very difficult to defend.

Continue to Revise Your Test Battery

You must revise your test battery continuously by improving, dropping, or adding tests. As new knowledge is available about standards, you also need to revise them along with any tables of norms you have compiled.

As new fitness tests (or new versions of tests) are published, you might consider replacing a test you are using with the improved version. For example, a straight-leg sit-up was used for many years in fitness test batteries. Students clasped their hands in back of the neck and performed the test with a straight back. In the last decade, this test was increasingly criticized because of its potential to create back problems. Several modifications have been proposed, the latest being a partial curl-up with the knees bent, performed to a cadence.

Sometimes we learn that a test does not measure the component of fitness we thought it did, and we must either find another test or use the test for the appropriate component. For instance, we believed for a long time that the sit-and-reach test measured low-back flexibility. Recent research has shown, however, that the test does not measure low-back flexibility but does measure hamstring flexibility. Thus, keeping up with the latest literature on fitness tests is important to maintaining an up-to-date test battery.

Develop Your Own Curricular Materials

As we said at the beginning of this book, fitness testing is only a small part of a fitness curriculum. Once you have identified the components of fitness you want to teach, develop units of instruction for each. For example, if you choose cardiorespiratory endurance as one of your fitness components, teach your students the factors that affect cardiorespiratory capacity. Older students can learn how to determine their target exercise heart rate and what variables of exercise (frequency, intensity, duration, and type of exercise) affect development of cardiorespiratory endurance. Even first graders can understand that the heart beats faster when they move faster.

Include a variety of sample activities in your lesson plans. Help your students understand that there are many ways to improve fitness by offering them varied opportunities for physical activity.

Be sure to stress the relationship between fitness and health. Young children may already show precursors to later heart disease. Despite lack of in-class time for vigorous physical exercise, you can teach students the importance of good fitness behaviors and encourage them to be active outside of class. You might even ask students to keep a log of such outside activities.

You also can encourage family participation in fitness activities. Hold a family fitness night at the school to focus on how families can exercise together.

Encourage children to ask their parents to exercise with them. Provide fitness-related handouts for children to take home to parents.

If time permits, you can expand your fitness curriculum to include areas such as nutrition and stress management. Students may learn something about nutrition in health class, but you can stress the relationship between nutrition and physical fitness. Teaching children the importance of healthy eating to control weight may help them avoid later weight problems. You can explain the value of exercise in stress management to students as well.

Develop Your Own Award System

The role of awards in promoting fitness is controversial. Some test developers believe awards are appropriate for children who have met designated standards of fitness, thinking that such awards motivate children to work for fitness. Others feel that awards can discourage students from trying to improve when they don't believe they can improve enough to win one.

Some test developers prefer to recognize participation in activities rather than attainment of certain levels of fitness. In such recognition systems, every child who participates receives a certificate and every child who is tested receives a sticker. Test results are used only to inform the child of his or her fitness status, not to determine awards.

If you want to give performance awards to children, you first have to decide what criteria are to be met in order to receive the award. If you have norm-referenced standards, you can use the percentile tables presented in Appendix C (Tables A.1-A.20) and choose a percentile cutoff for the award. Do you want to reward students who reach the 50th percentile? The 75th percentile? If you use criterion-referenced standards, you can use Tables A.21 to A.24 to set criteria for the awards.

Once you have determined the standards for your awards, then you must identify the type of award you want to give. Awards do not have to be expensive; a certificate handed out at an assembly is often sufficient. Inexpensive awards, such as pencils imprinted with the name of the school, might also be appropriate.

Summary

- The advantages to creating your own test battery include
  - choosing the components of fitness you think are most important,
  - tailoring your tests to your facilities or students, and
  - developing local standards.
- The disadvantages to creating your own test battery are
  - the lack of computer programs, curricular materials, or testing materials that come with national test batteries,
  - the need to revise the battery yourself continuously,
  - the need to create your own norms and standards, and
  - the need to develop your own award system and awards.
- Follow these seven steps to develop your own test battery:

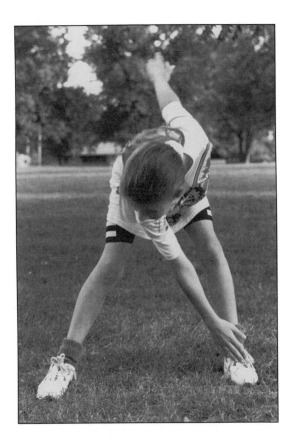

- Determine the important components of fitness.
- Select a test for each component.
- Try the test battery on a small group.
- Revise the test battery.
- Administer the revised test battery to the total group.
- Develop local norms and standards.
- Continue to revise your test battery.

- In your test battery, you may focus on a particular part of the body (to measure the flexibility or strength fitness component, for example) or measure a combination of health-related and performance-related aspects. Whatever you choose, make sure it reflects your definition of physical fitness.
- You may choose to select tests from different national batteries or to develop your own. If you develop your own, be sure to establish their validity and reliability.
- Prepare your test battery trial group as you would for any standard test. Use this trial to discover any problems in administering the tests.
- Revise your test battery on the basis of your trial experiences. Record in writing problems and changes in test procedures. If necessary, replace tests that don't work with others that measure the same components.
- Create appropriate scoring sheets and organize testing for your total group. Teach the students your testing system and allow them time to practice. Be sure to record scores in order to develop norms and standards. Don't compare results across tests if they are taken from different test batteries.

- To develop your own norms, collect several hundred scores for each age group and sex. Then develop a table of percentiles on computer and choose your standards. Health-related standards are very difficult to determine; your best option, if you wish to use them, is to find a test from a national test battery that is very similar to yours and use its standards.
- Continue to revise your test battery, norms, and standards. Keep up with developments in fitness testing so you can update your battery as new tests or versions of tests come out and as we learn more about what tests actually measure.
- Develop curricular materials that correspond to the fitness components you choose to teach. Provide a variety of fitness activities and stress the importance of good fitness behaviors. Encourage family fitness and, if you have the time, include additional areas of fitness such as nutrition and stress management.
- If you wish, develop your own award system. It can be based on participation or test performance. Select your award criteria and awards.

CHAPTER 6

Testing: Preparation, Administration, Recording, and Analysis

Cynthia Pemberton, PhD

Now that you've considered all the options and selected the fitness test battery that best suits your students and situation, half your job is done. The other half involves testing, interpreting, and using the results in your program.

Testing, to be accurate and beneficial for children, takes considerable preparation. It requires that you plan carefully so the testing procedure goes smoothly and safely, taking into account any special needs of your students. It also requires that students be prepared for the testing process. Do they know how to perform each test, and have they practiced it with good form? Do they understand the reasons for the testing and what each test measures? Are they afraid of testing or are they looking forward to it? And do they know what they will be expected to do and wear during testing?

How you administer the test can influence both the children's scores and their attitudes toward testing. How could you encourage your students' best performance? Do you know what details of testing will make the process easier and more accurate?

And once you get accurate test results, there is still the question of what to do with them. What's the optimal way to record, analyze, and summarize results?

This chapter will show you how to make the best use of the tests you've chosen while keeping your students interested and involved in the testing process. Let's begin with the first step—preparation.

Teacher Preparation

Advance preparation is key to successful testing. You will need to do the following before you ever schedule a test:

- Sequence the tests.
- Schedule and organize testing.
- Consider safety factors.
- Obtain necessary equipment.
- Design efficient scoring sheets.
- Locate and train assistants.

If you have children with special needs in your classes, you also should consider how you will accommodate them.

Test Sequence

Sequence the tests by the amount of exertion that they require. Give a cardiovascular test that requires maximal exertion by itself or, if that's not possible, at the end of the testing session. If given at the beginning, it will tire the students for subsequent tests. Also avoid giving several muscular strength or endurance tests during one session unless you allow plenty of time between tests for muscles to recover.

You can schedule together in one session tests that require submaximal effort or have short recovery times. For example, skinfold measurement, sit-ups, and flexibility testing could be completed during one testing period.

Test Scheduling and Site Organization

Test early in the school year and at the end of the year or semester, but not during the first few weeks of the year, because you will need to prepare students for testing. Do not test more frequently than 8 to 10 weeks apart, because less time is probably not enough for changes in fitness to become detectable.

Be sure to use the same tests, with the same procedures and in the same sequence, each time you test. Otherwise your results may not be comparable. In particular, only have one person do skinfold testing unless you have properly trained several people and checked them for between-tester reliability.

How you organize testing will probably be determined by time, facility, and equipment restraints and the number of assistants you have. Choose whether to administer all tests at once, group several tests, or use them one at a time; whether to test all students or smaller groups of students; and whether to test individually or through testing stations.

If your classes are small and you have enough equipment and assistants, you may choose to present all tests at once to all students. This traditional way to administer tests has some disadvantages. It is not an efficient use of class time because children may spend a lot of time waiting to be tested, and it requires that students put out a series of maximal efforts all at the same time.

One way to make this option more efficient is to use testing stations. To set up stations, mark off an area within the test site for each test you administer. Students move from one area to the next as they complete each test. For this system to work, you must teach students prior to testing how to perform the tests at each station and what they are to do during and between tests. Follow these steps:

1. Demonstrate the procedures for each test and have children practice them. Give younger children several opportunities to practice since they may not

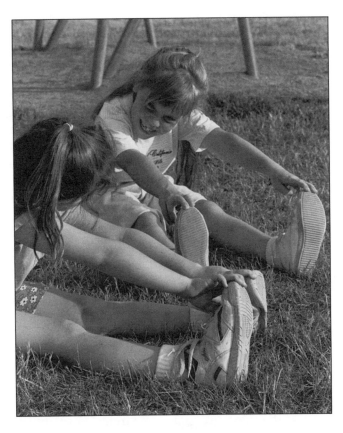

have had much experience in fitness testing. Older students will have had more experience and be better at remembering sequences of instructions.

2. Explain to students how to rotate from station to station and what to do as they wait to be tested. You may want to move younger children through stations in small groups, with each student sitting down before and after being tested. When the entire group has been tested, you or an assistant can take them as a group to the next station.

3. Reinforce your instructions by posting diagrams and key points for each test on bulletin boards in the gym, the locker room, or the classroom. Post a copy at each station during testing as well.

If skinfold measurement is part of the testing sequence, make sure that station provides privacy during testing. You can put up movable screens or locate the area somewhere far away from other students.

If your classes are large or your equipment or assistants are limited, you could test students in smaller groups, do only one or a few tests at a time, use testing stations for multiple tests, or test only a few students on a single test on a given day. For example, you could measure two or three students' body composition while the other students are doing warm-ups or another activity. The following class period you could test three more, and so on, until the entire class was finished. This would also provide you with more time to interact with students and make it easier to keep their test information private.

Whatever system you choose, be sure that all students go through it in the same order. If they don't their scores will not be comparable and cannot be summarized as a group.

Safety

To ensure the safety of students during testing, follow these guidelines:

- Give students opportunities to practice, younger students more than older ones. Make sure they are using proper form; correct them if they aren't.
- Ask students to wear nonrestrictive clothing and proper footwear for testing (see the section "Appropriate Dress" later in this chapter for details).
- Choose a test site that has enough space for all the students being tested and the equipment. If outdoors, make sure that the surface (grass, concrete, blacktop) is suitable for all tests. Whether testing is done indoors or out, provide mats for sit-ups and flexibility testing.
- Check all equipment prior to testing to ensure it is functioning properly.
- Check the test site prior to testing for possible hazards such as water, glass, or objects on the floor or ground or for potential interference from other students in the area (particularly when testing is done outside).
- Make sure the children know what your emergency procedures are, including what you will do in case of emergency, where to go if they are sent for assistance, and what to tell those they ask to assist.
- Monitor environmental conditions if cardiovascular testing is to be done outdoors. If the combined temperature and humidity values or pollution levels reach a dangerous point, reschedule testing.
- If testing outdoors, bad weather may force you to reschedule.
- Have students warm up with cardiovascular activity to increase their body temperature and then stretch to ready the muscles before each test.

Equipment

At the beginning of each year, check your equipment inventory. See how many of each piece of equipment you have, and check whether each is in good condition. You should have an adequate amount of mats, sit-and-reach boxes (or yardsticks for the V-sit), skinfold calipers, chinning bars (or modified pull-up test equipment), stopwatches, and traffic cones.

You can purchase all of this equipment or build the sit-and-reach boxes easily yourself. Don't spend a lot of money on calipers for skinfold measurement; inexpensive calipers are just as effective as the more expensive ones.

Scoring Sheets

Well-designed scoring sheets or cards make recording students' test scores more efficient. Each scoring sheet should include spaces for at least the following:

- Student's name, sex, age, and grade level
- Teacher's name
- Name of each test in the test battery
- Record of each trial for each test (check the directions for your fitness tests)

Additional spaces might be included for the goal score or criterion standard for each test and for pre- and posttest information.

You can choose to have a scoring sheet for each student or create a master scoring sheet for the test administrator. With individual scoring sheets, it's easier to record results for several years' testing. Students can also take the sheets with them from station to station. With a master scoring sheet, students don't have to handle any test results. (See Figure 6.1 for a sample individual scoring sheet and Figure 6.2 for a sample master scoring sheet.)

Another deciding factor might be whether the scores are to be taken off the sheets immediately and entered into a computer or whether other important information such as standards need to be added to the sheets. In the latter case, you might want the space on the individual sheets.

Student's name or identification number _____   Teacher's name _____

Testing date 1 _____   Age _____   Sex _____   Grade _____

Testing date 2 _____

Test item	Score test 1	Criterion standard	Standard met	Goal	Goal achieved	Score test 2	Criterion standard	Standard met	Goal	Goal achieved
1										
2										
3										
4										
5										

Recommendations: _____

Figure 6.1   Sample individual recording sheet.

Testing date 1 _____   Teacher's name _____

Testing date 2 _____   Grade _____

Student name or identification #	Sex	Age	Test item 1 Date / Criterion standard / Goal	Test item 2 Date / Criterion standard / Goal	Test item 3 Date / Criterion standard / Goal	Test item 4 Date / Criterion standard / Goal	Test item 5 Date / Criterion standard / Goal
Student 1			1	1	1	1	1
			2	2	2	2	2
Student 2			1	1	1	1	1
			2	2	2	2	2
Student 3			1	1	1	1	1
			2	2	2	2	2

*Circle criterion standard if met or exceeded.
**Circle goal if met or exceeded.

Figure 6.2   Sample group recording sheet.

Test Assistants

You can do testing more efficiently and effectively if you have assistants. But where do you find them? Parents would be a good choice, but many of them now work during the day. Try these possibilities:

- Local college or university students
- Retired individuals
- Volunteers from companies, hospitals, or civic organizations
- Older students who are teachers' aides

All assistants, regardless of their prior experience in administering fitness tests, should go through a training session before they assist. This training should identify possible problems in test administration, such as not following testing procedures exactly. Review all testing procedures carefully, even if you administer the same tests yearly. Train individuals without prior test administration experience even more thoroughly than those with it. Training should include

- an overview of what each test measures,
- specific procedures for each test,
- details on how tests will be administered,
- opportunities to practice test procedures, and
- an evaluation of each assistant's testing skills.

If it's not possible to train some of the assistants to do testing, you can still use their help. They can watch over students who are waiting to be tested and keep students from comparing scores or teasing each other. They can help record scores and, when self-testing is used, check that students are using proper form. And finally, they can offer encouragement and congratulations to children to enhance test performance and make testing more enjoyable.

Testing Children With Special Needs

In your classes you may have children with various disabilities: sensory (deafness or blindness), mental (Down syndrome or mental retardation), or physical (muscular dystrophy or missing limbs). Despite the disability, physical fitness is as important for these students as it is for your other students. Fitness not only helps them prevent diseases due to a sedentary lifestyle but also enhances their ability to perform physical tasks and provides opportunities for social interaction with nondisabled children.

Assessing abilities is important in developing special programs for children with disabilities, yet most of the time standardized tests won't work for them. The test items don't fit their needs, and the results cannot be directly compared to standard norms. Accurately testing these children requires additional information and effort on your part.

Difficulties in following the usual test protocols include these:

- *Ability:* Some students will be physically unable to perform the tests in the manner prescribed. You may find that making slight modifications or providing some assistance will allow students to successfully participate, but this runs some risk of jeopardizing the test's validity.

- *Understanding:* The student may not be capable of understanding or following the test instructions as they are written. You may need to offer verbal or physical guidance to convey the information.
- *Motivation:* Because they are discouraged, embarrassed, or frustrated, or because they don't comprehend the idea of "doing your best," some of these students won't give their best effort during testing. You have to discover ways to encourage them to participate fully.
- *Experience:* These students may not have had much fitness testing experience. Many concepts may be new to them, so you may need to take extra time to explain and practice testing and to reassure them.

A good approach to considering how to adapt testing to children with special needs is to ask yourself these questions:

- How does testing relate to program objectives?
- How should I prepare myself for testing?
- How should I prepare the student for testing?
- How should I prepare the test site for this student?
- What will be done with the test scores?

Let's talk briefly about each one.

Testing and Program Objectives

You should always relate testing to your program's objectives, but the objectives for children with special needs may differ from those for the rest of your class. To do a good job of setting those objectives, you must know the effects of the child's disabilities on physical performance. You also should consider whether the objectives you choose are ones that will improve the child's quality of life. Being able to run faster may not benefit the child much, while being able to lift a certain amount of weight or stretch a particular distance might help him or her function more effectively in daily life.

Preparing Yourself for Testing

To test properly, you must be knowledgeable about each individual student's abilities and about the test battery. Knowing about the general effects of a disability is a first step, but individual children's abilities will vary considerably. For instance, visual impairment can mean total blindness, partial sight, or a more specific problem, like difficulty tracking a moving object. Even within partial sight, there are individual gradations: Can the child see only moving objects? How clearly can the child see detail?

Add to that what you know about the test you plan to use. Can you adjust it to fit that particular child? Would a protocol meant for a younger child be suitable? Or should a completely different test be chosen?

Whatever test you select should be sensitive enough for the child to achieve some score and demonstrate improvement. For example, a child unable to do a bent arm hang because of lack of strength might measure arm strength by lifting a dumbbell. Or, if you measure an endurance run by laps completed, then measure not only full laps but quarter or half laps. There will be improvement even if the child only runs slightly more the next time. Another alternative is to note how well a movement is performed rather than the number of times it is performed, again to show progress toward the goal. It's important to look at the quality of a movement before being concerned about the number of times the movement can be repeated, especially when it is first being learned.

Preparing Your Student for Testing

How you prepare a student depends on that student's particular disability. If the person has a learning disability, you may need to create special hand cues or picture signs; if the person is blind, you may need to add some auditory signals. Keep in mind that adaptations you make for children with disabilities may actually be helpful to your entire class, as long as those changes don't change the reliability or validity of the test.

Make sure each student understands the testing protocols and performance strategies such as pacing. Before testing, clarify everything again, and have them practice under test conditions.

It's also important that you have a good rapport with the children before testing, as the test situation may be threatening. Try to keep testing fun and not too serious.

Preparing Your Test Site

It's likely you will have to modify standard tests to help students perform. For example, a child who can't do a sit-up alone may be able to if someone holds her hand. Or to time a run for a blind child you may need to replace a digital timer with one that buzzes. In situations like these, be sure to have the necessary people or equipment present.

Ensuring good test results also means paying attention to emotional and cognitive performance barriers as well as physical ones. For instance, a child with a behavior disorder may need to be tested in an isolated space, away from distractions, with the test area marked more clearly. For all children with special needs, check for distractions that might interfere with testing.

If the children with special needs that you work with have low fitness, they probably tire easily. To get a better sense of their abilities, spread testing out over time instead of doing it all at once.

Using the Test Scores

Interpreting test scores for children with disabilities is challenging. Most test standards are developed on children without disabilities; there aren't yet a lot of good databases on those with disabilities (see the resource list at the end of the chapter for possible sources for databases). If you can't find a valid database, it's probably better to focus on whether the student improves over time.

Also, scores may not truly reflect a child's capabilities if the test circumstances hindered performance. A blind child who had to run around a track with the assistance of a trained runner as a guide may not have performed optimally. This is not an excuse; we make adjustments for all children when we take into account whether it was very hot, or rainy and muddy, on the test day.

To best assist the child with disabilities, you should observe the testing and take notes. Then when you examine the results, you can check to see whether performance might have been affected by outside circumstances. Also consider your experience with the child. During activities, does the child keep up with

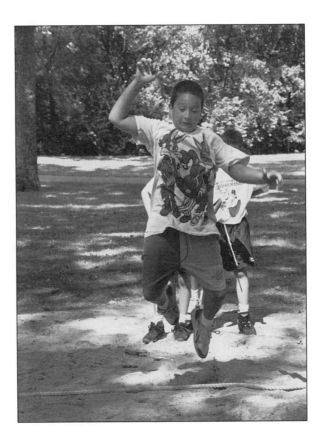

the others? Have you seen him or her successfully perform in class what was failed in the test?

As with test results for any children, be sure to help students with disabilities understand what their results mean. Examine your program based on test results and see how you can revise it to help them improve. Coming full circle to where we started, use the test results to assess if you are meeting your program objectives.

To learn more about fitness testing for children with special needs, refer to the resource list at the end of this chapter.

Student Preparation

Test is a word that can strike fear into the hearts of children. Being evaluated can be a bit scary, but if you prepare your students properly, they can find it to be interesting and fun, while you can achieve more accurate assessments. You need to get them ready for testing, both physically and mentally; here are some ideas on how to do it.

Physical Readiness

Students must practice performing tests prior to testing if you are to get a true picture of their abilities. It's hard to get a reasonable assessment of what children can do if they are struggling with how to move.

Before students practice, demonstrate each test, even if they have taken the test before. Students may not remember the procedures clearly, or the testing protocol may have changed. When you demonstrate, show students common errors made during each test.

Give students sufficient time to practice, especially younger students. As for any physical activity, students should warm up and stretch before practicing. Teach students a stretching routine at least 5 min long that they can use for this purpose. As they practice, monitor for errors in form and help correct those errors. Form is particularly important for sit-ups, pull-ups, running, and the sit-and-reach test. Make sure students follow the test procedures exactly as outlined in the test directions.

For those tests that require it, such as the mile run, sit-ups, or pull-ups, focus on teaching students pacing. For running, Corbin and Pangrazi (1989) suggest using traffic cones to teach the concept of pacing. Ask students to attempt to take the same number of running steps between cones at approximately the same speed. Also try having students run short distances, such as a quarter of a mile, first as fast as possible and then slower, taking twice the amount of time. Another way to teach pacing is to beat a drum or set a metronome as they practice so they can move to the beat.

Finally, if testing students for cardiovascular endurance, make sure they have a chance to participate in plenty of aerobic activities. Some additional suggestions for fitness testing reported in the National Children and Youth Fitness studies (Ross, Dotson, Katz, Errecart, & Gaines, 1985; Ross & Gilbert, 1985; Ross & Pate, 1987) are included in the next section, "Test Administration."

In the past, the wisdom of allowing students to practice before a test has been questioned because of concern that test items might be interpreted as the only way to achieve fitness goals. Just because sit-ups are included in testing doesn't mean that abdominal strength and endurance should be built only by doing sit-ups. Teach students a variety of ways to accomplish this and other fitness goals.

Mental Readiness

The first step in preparing students mentally for fitness testing is to talk not about testing but about basic physical fitness concepts. Students need to understand why they are being tested and what the results mean for them if they are to feel involved in testing. Most of the major fitness testing programs emphasize the importance of fitness education and have developed related curricular materials for physical education teachers.

Once students have this background information, you can describe and demonstrate each test. Encourage students to ask questions during the demonstrations to clarify testing procedures. Afterward, post key points of each test around the gym.

Talk with students about what they can expect to feel physically during testing. They should know which feelings are normal and which mean they should stop. For example, during a running test children's mouths and throats often become dry. This is a normal response. But students should stop if they

- become dizzy or disoriented,
- develop difficulty in breathing (wheeze or cough violently),

- stop sweating,
- become pale, or
- exhibit any signs of heat illness (headache, nausea, cramps).

It is important that children be aware of these physical cues, as many fitness tests are maximal tests that require a paced effort.

After students have had a chance to practice the tests, ask them to set goals for the score they would like to attain on each test (for more on goal setting, see "Setting Goals With Children", p. 102). Have them consider how well they did on previous tests and decide how much they can improve. Be sure to let students know how and when they will get testing results.

Encourage students to perform their best when being tested, emphasizing that their best effort on these tests will give them the most realistic picture of their physical fitness level. Ask them to encourage each other during testing. Pairing students so one student can coach as the other is being tested is sometimes helpful. Be sure to make it clear that students will not be allowed to ridicule others and that you will keep test scores confidential.

Appropriate Dress

Before testing, tell your students what tests you will do and what they should wear. In general, they should wear nonrestrictive clothing such as shorts, T-shirts, athletic socks, and some type of tennis shoe. If running is part of testing, a running shoe would be preferable to a basketball shoe. Warn students not to wear new shoes on test day, as the shoes may cause blisters. If you will take skinfold measurements, they should wear nonrestrictive clothing so you can reach the sites easily.

Test Administration

Now that you have prepared your students for testing and made arrangements for a test site, it is time to get yourself ready for what happens during the test. We have some tips on administering particular test procedures, but we also want to stress the importance of what you do and say to motivate children to do their best during testing.

Tips for Testing

For all tests, you must check the test site to ensure that the equipment and the site are organized and ready for use. By now you should be familiar with all test procedures, and during testing you should focus on monitoring students for proper performance of the tests.

To help you with some specific types of tests—running, sit-and-reach, sit-ups, pull-ups, and skinfold testing—here are some suggestions (Ross et al., 1985):

Running Tests

1. To prevent inaccurate lap counting, pair students into running and resting partners. Have the resting partner be responsible for counting the running student's laps. Supply pencil and paper for tallying the laps.

2. Measure your running track with a measuring wheel for exact distances, since many tracks are not a standard distance.

3. When administering this test to younger students, secure the assistance of a parent aide or another teacher. The assistant can help monitor the students.

4. When using the mile test, set a maximum of eight laps so that scoring will be manageable and so that the students will not be crowded as they run.

5. Use a digital stopwatch to prevent errors in scoring. You may want to have a backup one as well, in case the original malfunctions.

6. Remind students to tie their shoes before beginning the run.

Sit-and-Reach

1. Don't allow students to bend their knees during this test. Some test instructions direct the test administrator to lay a hand and lower arm lightly across the knees, which serves as a reminder to the student to keep the knees straight.

2. If the measuring scale includes a movable sliding block, don't permit students to flick the block beyond their reach.

3. Don't permit jerky movements, as they can lead to injury and inaccurate scores.

4. Require students to put their heads down during the stretch and reach full extension.

Sit-Ups

1. Demonstrate the following common errors to students before they begin practicing sit-ups: lifting the hips or buttocks off the mat as they sit up; lifting the elbows away from the chest; bringing the head back; and sitting up with a straight back rather than a curl.

2. During testing, group the students in threes, with one serving as an observer and the other holding the feet (if this follows your test's protocol).

3. Require students to move up to the specified position for completing the up portion of the sit-up, then down to the designated completion position.

4. Require the feet and buttocks to be on the same surface.

5. Monitor body position during the sit-up and require students to maintain proper distance between the hips and the feet. Placing tape on the mat can act as a guide to students.

6. To help prevent back injury, provide a soft surface on which students can practice and perform the test.

Pull-Ups

1. Ask students to dry their hands before attempting pull-ups or flexed arm hangs. Wipe the bar clean before the attempt and allow students to apply gymnastics chalk (if available and acceptable under your test's protocol).

2. Demonstrate common errors, such as swinging, bouncing, head thrown back, and bent arms before students practice.

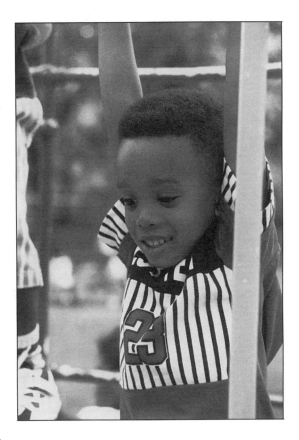

Skinfold Testing

1. Practice taking skinfold measurements before testing takes place.

2. Provide a reasonable degree of privacy for the student during testing.

3. Check the calibration of the calipers periodically.

4. Refrain from joking with the student during testing.

5. Properly locate and mark all skinfold sites.

6. Place a mark on the floor for students to stand on and one on the wall for them to look at during triceps skinfold measurement. This keeps students in proper position.

7. Stand directly behind the student's right arm when taking the triceps skinfold.

8. Shake the student's arm before taking the triceps skinfold to help relax the arm.

9. If measuring the triceps on younger students, have them step up onto a table, chair, or folded mat to be at your level. This prevents you having to bend over constantly during testing.

10. For the calf skinfold, have students place their right foot onto a chair, mat, or table so that their bent knee forms a 90-degree angle.

11. Do not repeat sets of three measurements until they fall within 2 mm, and do not take more than seven measurements at a site. Stop as soon as any three consecutive measures fall within 2 mm; if they don't, use the median of all seven measurements as the student's score.

12. Alternate taking skinfolds between one site and another, such as the triceps and calf.

Motivating Students

For some students, physical fitness testing is a threat to their self-worth. When they feel this way, students often protect themselves by putting out less effort so they can blame poor test performance on not trying their hardest.

To counteract these feelings of threat, help students feel they are competent (Harter, 1980) and can succeed in fitness testing. You can do this by providing students with a supportive learning and testing environment.

Always encourage students to put forth their best effort and never belittle their performance. Give students opportunities to set goals for testing. Talk to them individually when possible; say "John, I know you can reach your goal on this sit-up test, try your best" or "Sally, you've been working on your running so hard, let's see you meet your goal on this mile run." You also can use a buddy system that gives each student a classmate for encouragement throughout testing.

Never compare students with each other (Roberts, 1992), saying "I bet Timmy can do more sit-ups than you" or "I don't think anyone can beat the school record in pull-ups." Some teachers feel this will motivate students, but more students are discouraged than are motivated; it creates unnecessary anxiety for students, who then think they should compare themselves with others. Also, don't single out students to perform in front of others; this may either embarrass the chosen students or cause them to show off, which indirectly makes other students feel less competent. Instead ask students to challenge themselves to better their own past scores.

Always discourage teasing and ridicule among students but especially when working with children who are obese. Such children often find fitness testing to be a horrible experience because of classmates' comments. Give children who are obese special attention to alleviate their anxiety and show support for putting forth a best effort. If they refuse to participate, allow participation at another time when they feel more comfortable. It's important to be responsive to these children, as they are aware of their obesity and may feel threatened by fitness testing.

You also may use self-testing to enhance motivation for testing, reinforce correct test procedures, and help students (particularly older ones) learn fitness concepts. Most current fitness tests are not very complex and are suitable for students' use. Even skinfold testing, which requires special skills, can be performed accurately by students with proper training and experience (Whitehead, Frey, & Corbin, 1989; Whitehead, Parker, & Pemberton, 1992). Allowing students to self-test gives them a sense of control, and it also reinforces the importance of proper testing procedures.

Self-testing lends itself to a station format, in which students move from station to station performing each test on their own. You can develop checklists for doing each test and allow partners or groups of three students to practice the tests. In groups of three, one student takes the test; one administers the test by counting, keeping time, or measuring; and the third uses the checksheet to make sure testing is performed correctly. Other activities such as tumbling can be going on in the gym as testing goes on, which keeps all students active and prevents them from waiting in line. If you already designate some class time for free choice of activities, self-testing might be a choice on a specific day.

Recording and Analyzing Results

The mechanical aspects of testing—recording and analyzing data—are important but easy to overlook. It's crucial to record and enter data as accurately as possible for feedback to students; it's also worth thinking about what types of analysis would give the best information to students, parents, and school administrators.

If you have a computer program for data analysis, you'll have to go through the tedious job of entering the data. If you're lucky enough to find someone to assist you, be sure to spot check the printout of scores against a sample of the scores on the score sheets. If you find a lot of errors, re-enter the data.

If computer software accompanies the fitness test you use, an analysis of the data is probably available at the push of a key. If you don't have ready-made software, you have two choices: either have the computer expert in your district develop a program to calculate and analyze results, or describe the test results in some simple ways that are easy to calculate manually.

Three ways to analyze data that don't require a computer are calculating the average, the median, and the standard deviation or an interpercentile range.

- Compute the *average* by adding all of the student's scores together and dividing by the number of students tested. (The average can also be called the mean.)
- For the *median*, find the middle of the distribution for the scores. The median score is the score that half of the scores are above and half below.
- Calculate the *standard deviation* (which is the deviation of scores from the mean) or the *interpercentile range* (an even range of scores either side of the 50th percentile, usually from 75 to 25).

To find the standard deviation, use the following formula:

$$SD = \sqrt{\frac{\Sigma x^2 - \frac{(\Sigma x)^2}{N}}{N}}$$

SD = standard deviation
x = each student's test score
Σ = add
N = number of students who have scores
Σx^2 = square each student's test score and then
 add all of the squared scores together
$(\Sigma x)^2$ = add all of the students' test scores
 together and then square that number

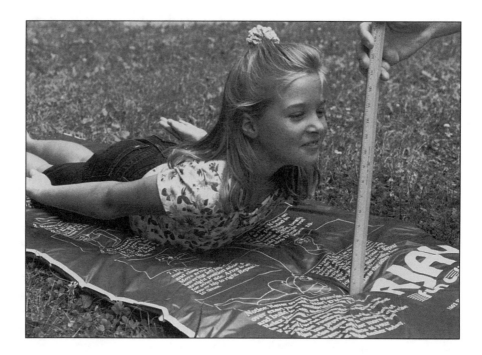

Be sure to include in your analysis information about the number of students who meet the criterion-referenced standards. Information on norms is less helpful because it compares children to each other rather than addressing the importance of the results to children's health.

When you report fitness testing scores and analysis to school administrators and parents, thoroughly explain what the numbers represent. Presenting trends or patterns for groups of students is usually most informative, using overheads or handouts that show class means, ranges, and standard deviations compared to criterion standards or national norms. You also can compare results across years or show how many children reached their personal goals. In addition you could share test results from the cognitive and motor skills areas, mentioning circumstances of your physical education program that influence these results or may affect future improvement of test scores, such as time, facilities, equipment, or curriculum. Presenting test results is an opportunity to educate the community about fitness and its role in the physical education curriculum.

Summary

- Sequence tests by the amount of exertion they require so test results are not affected by students' tiredness.
- Schedule testing at the beginning and end of the year or semester. Use the same tests in the same sequence and with the same procedures each time.
- Depending on your circumstances, choose whether to administer all tests at once, group tests, or administer them one at a time; whether to test all students or smaller groups of students; and whether to test individually or through testing stations.
- Follow these steps for using testing stations:

- Demonstrate and have students practice the procedures.
- Explain to students how to rotate from station to station and what to do while waiting.
- Reinforce your instructions by posting diagrams and key points for each test.

- For safety, make sure the students are prepared for testing, the test site and equipment are free from hazards, and the weather is suitable if testing is done outdoors. Always have students warm up before testing.
- At the beginning of the year, check that you have enough equipment in good condition for testing.
- Design an effective individual or master scoring sheet for your test battery.
- Find and train test assistants who can aid you in administering tests or supervising children during testing.
- Be aware that children with special needs may have difficulties with the usual test protocols due to a lack of ability, understanding, motivation, or experience.
- Adapt testing for children with special needs by considering these questions:

  - How does testing relate to program objectives?
  - How should I prepare myself for testing?
  - How should I prepare the student for testing?
  - How should I prepare the test site for this student?
  - What will be done with the test scores?

- Prepare your students physically and mentally for testing, and tell them what to wear.
- During testing, keep test procedures in mind. Don't forget to encourage students, and don't compare students to each other as a way to motivate them. Be particularly careful to support children who are obese.
- When possible, allow children to do self-testing. It gives them a sense of control and reinforces proper test procedures.
- When an assistant enters test scores, be sure to spotcheck the entries for accuracy.
- If you don't have software to analyze test results, ask a computer expert in your district to develop such software, or calculate some analyses manually. Three possible analyses are the average, the median, and the standard deviation or interpercentile range.
- When you report fitness test scores and analyses to school administrators and parents, explain what the numbers mean. Present trends within groups and over time, and comparisons with criterion standards or national norms. Mention the circumstances of your physical education program that might influence test results, now or in the future.

References

Corbin, C., & Pangrazi, R. (1989) *Teaching strategies for improving fitness*. Dallas: Cooper Institute for Aerobics Research.

Harter, S. (1980). The development of competence motivation in the mastery of cognitive and physical skills: Is there still a place for joy? In G.C. Roberts and D.M. Landers (Eds.), *Psychology of motor behavior and sport* (pp. 3-29). Champaign, IL: Human Kinetics.

Roberts, G. (Ed.) (1992). *Motivation in sport and exercise.* Champaign, IL: Human Kinetics.

Ross, J.G., Dotson, C.O., Katz, S.J., Errecart, M.T., & Gaines, G. (1985). *Final report: National children and youth fitness study.* (Contract No. 282-82-0059). Washington, DC: Office of Disease Prevention and Health Promotion.

Ross, J.G., & Gilbert, G.G. (1985). The national children and youth fitness study: A summary of findings. *Journal of Physical Education, Recreation and Dance.* **56**, 45-50.

Ross, J.G., & Pate, R.S. (1987). The national children and youth fitness study II: A summary of findings. *Journal of Physical Education, Recreation and Dance,* **58**, 51-61.

Whitehead, J.R., Frey, M., & Corbin, C.B. (1989, April). *Self-testing of physical fitness: The accuracy of skinfold measures taken by children.* Paper presented at the meeting of the American Alliance for Health, Physical Education, Recreation and Dance, Boston.

Whitehead, J.R., Parker, M.A., & Pemberton, C.L. (1992, April). *Fitness tests as opportunities for cognitive learning: An experiment using skinfold testing.* Paper presented at the meeting of the American Alliance for Health, Physical Education, Recreation and Dance, Indianapolis.

Resources for Children With Special Needs

Publications

American Alliance for Health, Physical Education and Recreation (1975). *Testing for impaired, disabled, and handicapped individuals.* Reston, VA: AAHPERD Publications.

Auxter, D., & Pyfer, J. (1989). *Principles and methods of adapted physical education and recreation.* St. Louis: Times Mirror/Mosby.

Eichstaedt, C.B., & Lavay, B.W. (1992). *Physical activity for individuals with mental retardation: Infancy through adulthood.* Champaign, IL: Human Kinetics.

Folio, M.R. (1986). *Physical education programming for exceptional learners.* Rockville, MD: Aspen

Jansma, P. (Ed.) (1988). *The psychomotor domain and the seriously handicapped* (3rd ed.). Lantham, MD: University Press of America.

Johnson, R.E., & Lavay, B. (1989). Fitness testing for children with special needs: An alternative approach. *Journal of Physical Education, Recreation and Dance,* **60**(6), 50-53.

Lavay, B., Reid, G., & Cressler-Chaviz, M. (1990). Measuring the cardiovascular endurance of persons with mental retardation: A critical review. In K. Pandolf (Ed.), *Exercise science sport review* (pp. 263-290). Baltimore: Williams & Wilkins.

Miles, B.H., Nierengarden, M.E., & Nearing, R.J. (1988). A review of the eleven most often cited assessment instruments used in adapted physical education. *Clinical Kinesiology,* 42, 33-31.

Moon, M.S., & Renzaglia, A. (1982). Physical fitness and the mentally retarded: A critical review of the literature. *Journal of Special Education*, **16**, 125-132.

Oded, B. (1983). *Pediatric sports medicine for the practitioner: From physiologic principles to clinical adaptations*. New York: Springer-Verlag.

Seaman, J.A., & DePauw, K.P. (1989). *The new adapted physical education: A developmental approach*. Palo Alto, CA: Mayfield.

Shephard, R.J. (1990). *Fitness in special populations*. Champaign, IL: Human Kinetics.

Sherrill, C. (1993). *Adapted physical education and recreation: A multidisciplinary approach* (4th ed.). Dubuque, IA: Brown.

Short, F.X. (1990). Measurement and appraisal. In J.P. Winnick (Ed.), *Adapted physical education and sport* (pp. 51-69). Champaign, IL: Human Kinetics.

Werder, J., & Kalakian, L. (1985). *Assessment in adapted physical education*. Minneapolis: Burgess.

TESTS*

Alabama Special Olympics Fitness Battery

Roswal, Floyd, Roswal, Jessup, Pass, Klecka, Montelione, Vaccaro, & Dunleavy. (1985).
Available from G. Roswell, Jacksonville State University, Department of Physical Education, Jacksonville, AL 36265

The test manual includes normative physical fitness data based on a sample of 2,084 Alabama Special Olympians, ages 8 to 68 years; measurements for 12 commonly used physical fitness items (except cardiovascular endurance); and norm-referenced tables by sex and age groups.

Kansas Adapted/Special Physical Education Test Manual

Johnson, R.E., & Lavay, B. (1988).
Available from Janet Wilson, Specialist in Physical Education, Kansas State Department of Education, 120 SE 10th St., Topeka, KS 66612

Included in this manual is Good's Health Related Physical Fitness Test/Kansas Revision. Pat Good (Special/Adapted Physical Education Specialist for Students With Mental Retardation, Howe School, 1800 Oakwood Blvd., Dearborn, MI 48124) originally developed the test procedures and has used them since 1981. They were revised and field tested in 1988 by a group of Kansas certified adapted physical education specialists. The health-related fitness test items included in this test are sit-ups, sit-and-reach, isometric push-ups and a bench press, and aerobic movement. The aerobic movement is a unique method of assessing cardiovascular endurance. The individuals ambulate in any fashion possible (e.g., briskly walking, running, propelling themselves in wheelchairs) while maintaining a pulse rate from 140 to 180 beats per minute for 12 min after a 6-min warm-up. The individual's pulse rate is monitored every 3 min during testing.

Physical Fitness and Motor Skill Levels of Individuals with Mental Retardation: Mild, Moderate, and Individuals with Down Syndrome: Ages 6 to 21

Eichstaedt, C.B., Wang, P.Y., Polacek, J.J., & Dohrmann, P.F. (1991).
Available from Dr. Jerry Polacek, Department of HPERD, Illinois State University, Normal, IL 61790-5120

The test battery includes 14 tests that measure the physical fitness and motor performance of persons with mental retardation from 6 to 21 years of age. Norms were established by testing over 4,000 persons with mental retardation from Illinois schools and agencies. This is one of the few norm-referenced tests to develop normative data with separate categories of mental retardation.

Physical Fitness Testing of the Disabled: Project UNIQUE

Winnick, J.P., & Short, Francis X. (1985).
Available from Human Kinetics, P.O. Box 5076, Champaign, IL 61825-5076.

This fitness test for youth from 10 to 17 is designed for both those who have sensory or orthopedic disabilities and those who don't. Test items cover body composition, muscular strength and endurance, flexibility, and cardiorespiratory endurance. The tester selects a classification for each individual tested, and that classification determines which subset of test items is administered. Norms for each classification appear in the appendixes. Besides the test instructions, the manual includes training information for those with disabilities covering a system for training, general fitness training guidelines, special considerations based on specific disabilities, and recommended activities and modifications of sports.

The Project Transition Assessment System

Jansma, Decker, Ersing, McCubbin, & Combs. (1988).
Available from Dr. Paul Jansma, The Ohio State University, Department of Physical Education, 343 Larkin Hall, Columbus, OH 43210

This assessment system includes both qualitative and quantitative measures of the following physical fitness items: sit-ups, bench press, sit-and-reach, grip strength, and 300-yd run/walk. All fitness items were determined to have functional value for individuals with mental retardation, including those with severe mental retardation, however, the measure of cardiovascular endurance is questionable. The system includes a unique qualitative format of scoring by measuring such factors as task completion, level of necessary prompting, and reinforcement strategies.

---

*Note. From *Physical Activity for Individuals With Mental Retardation: Infancy Through Adulthood* (pp. 101-103) by C.B. Eichstaedt and B.W. Lavay, Champaign, IL: Human Kinetics Publishers. Copyright 1992 by Carl B. Eichstaedt and Barry W. Lavay. Adapted by permission.

CHAPTER 7

Use of Test Results

Cynthia Pemberton, PhD

You've put forth a lot of effort to get good test results. Now it's time to use those results to

- make students aware of their fitness status,
- guide students to set appropriate goals for fitness,
- reward students who reach fitness goals or maintain good fitness behaviors,
- assess the quality of the physical education program and make changes, and
- evaluate student progress.

The key to using test results wisely is to keep them in perspective. They can be good motivators and measuring sticks when seen as general guidelines, but they should not be used to judge or discourage children or as the sole determinants of program content. With this in mind, let's talk about giving feedback to students.

Feedback

As we stated in chapter 1, testing is only part of the larger process of fitness education; but it is the part that focuses on what fitness means to the individual student. Because of that, it can catch students' (and parents') interest and motivate the student to become more fit.

If test results are to motivate, you must communicate them with sensitivity and confidentiality and relate them to fitness education. It also helps to use results to seek parents' support, as parents can greatly affect whether children decide to develop and continue healthy behaviors.

To make fitness testing results meaningful, share them with the students, and explain them. Present results as soon as possible after completing testing, and give results for all tests at the same time so one area of physical fitness is not emphasized over another. Give each student a written copy of his or her own fitness results with both verbal and written explanations of what those scores mean, especially in relation to some standard, criterion, or norm. Tell students which areas they have done well in and which they need to improve.

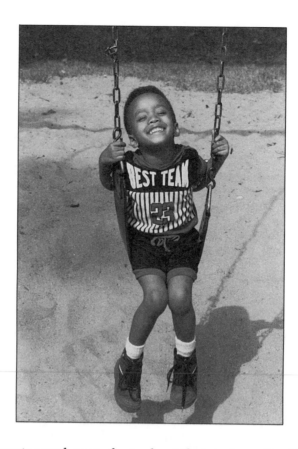

You may choose to speak to students about their test results either individually or in a group. Individual meetings are most desirable but often aren't possible because of time constraints. If they are willing, classroom teachers might meet with each child to review the results. Younger children may require more individual time since they aren't as familiar with testing and testing concepts. Give younger children simple explanations. For example, to a young child who needs to work on muscle strength alone, you might say: "Tammy, it looks like your physical fitness levels are great in all areas except one, and that is the area of muscle strength. In order to get stronger you'll have to do some activities where you push and pull with your arms. Let's see if we can think of some that you could do almost every day." Older children, who have participated in testing often and who grasp the basic principles of fitness, are better able to discuss results as a group. Any group discussion should cover only basic fitness information and the overall group's performance, *not* individuals' scores.

Give written feedback at the reading level of the children; ask a classroom teacher for help with developing materials if you aren't sure what's appropriate. For young children who can't read, you may have to create symbols to represent each fitness component (such as a running person for cardiovascular fitness) and the students' level (such as a smiley face for good performance).

Sensitivity and Confidentiality

Many students are self-conscious about their performance on physical fitness tests. To avoid embarrassing them, you should always present individual scores and their interpretation in written form *only* to that individual. Word the feedback in a nonthreatening way, but be truthful about whether the child's performance was acceptable and, if not, what he or she might do to improve it. Make specific comments on each area of fitness.

You also must watch that assistants or other children not reveal anyone's test scores. From the beginning, tell students that their scores are only for their information and not to be discussed with each other. No student has the right to know another's test scores, and no one should pressure another child into telling his or her scores. Also instruct all testing assistants to keep test results confidential.

To ensure confidentiality, store scoring sheets and test reports in a locked file drawer or cabinet. If you think a problem with security might occur, you can assign each student an identification number that only you and the student know. Use that number, rather than the student's name, to identify test materials. If sheets or reports are lost or stolen, students' identities are still safe.

Relating Results to Fitness Education

Once students have received their test results, talk with them as soon as possible about how they can improve those results. Focus not so much on how they did this time, but on what to do for next time. This is a good opportunity to teach children the skills they will need throughout life to stay fit.

Start by reviewing general fitness concepts, including the training principles of frequency, intensity, time (FIT), and type of exercise. Talk about what types of activities are best for each component of fitness. Then ask students to plan their individualized exercise and fitness prescription, based on their test results. As students plan, you can tell them more about the additional training concepts of overload, progression, and specificity. Some testing software supplies information tying test results to lifestyle change recommendations for your students. (For more on setting individual exercise goals, see "Setting Goals With Children" later in this chapter.)

Informing and Involving Parents

Parents and guardians are naturally concerned about their children's fitness. Reporting test results to them can help make them partners in promoting children's health.

Before testing, inform parents about the type of fitness testing to be done, its purpose, and the kind of feedback they and their child will receive. Stress that scores will be handled confidentially and that the testing procedures have been designed to make testing a positive experience. (See Figure 7.1 for a sample note to parents.)

After fitness testing, send all parents written information about their child's scores. Be sure to include materials that explain fitness basics and the meaning of the test results, and ask parents to discuss the results with their children at home. If children have set fitness goals based on their test results, give parents a copy of those goals.

When possible, schedule conferences with parents to discuss results. Before conferences begin, let all parents know that what is said during conferences

Dear Parents/Guardian:

We will be doing physical fitness testing at Brown Middle School throughout the school year during our physical education class time. We will be testing the areas of health-related physical fitness by asking your child to participate in several types of tests. Some of these tests will require little physical exertion, while others will require considerable effort. Your child will have the opportunity to practice each test beforehand so that he or she is familiar with the test.

The tests will be given so that all children are encouraged to do their best and competition between children is minimized. Your child's test results will not be shared with anyone but you and your child.

After all testing has been completed we will provide you and your child with written results. The test results will be discussed with your child and we would like to discuss your child's test results with you at our Back to School Night in May. We are also available to answer any questions you might have about the area of fitness and what fitness test results mean. We hope you will join us in encouraging your child to maintain a healthy level of physical fitness and to adopt good lifestyle behaviors to ensure a positive quality of life for now and in the future. If you have questions please call [phone no.].

Thank you! Keep moving!

Figure 7.1 Sample note to parents prior to testing.

will be kept confidential. Keep in mind that many parents hold misperceptions about the reasons for fitness testing, and they may feel sensitive about their own fitness status. Many also had negative experiences with physical education and testing when they went to school.

During conferences, present all of the test results, not overemphasizing one aspect but talking about the relationship of all the components of physical fitness to each other and to health. Educate parents about fitness, starting with a one-page general description of each fitness component (see Figure 7.2 for sample handout). Tell parents that they may contact you later if they have questions about the test results, and either give them a phone number to call or an opportunity to schedule an additional conference time, or do this in a follow-up letter.

One fitness component that parents often are confused about is body composition. Define body composition and explain to parents why a leaner body composition is desirable for health, then allow them to ask questions. Some people believe that if children's body composition is tested, children may develop eating disorders. There is no evidence for this belief. For their present and future health, children need accurate information about body composition and how they can maintain or change it.

If individual parent conferences cannot be scheduled, consider offering a presentation on physical fitness that includes distribution of students' physical fitness test results. Be sure the presentation is balanced, not overemphasizing one aspect of physical fitness more than another.

Educating parents and the community about fitness can be done on a year-round basis. Petray (1990) has some suggestions for educational activities:

- Hold a physical fitness night at the school. Students can demonstrate activities that develop each of the components of fitness, and you can describe not only the fitness aspect of your physical education program but the cognitive and motor skill aspects as well.

Health-related fitness consists of five components:

- Cardiovascular fitness
- Body composition
- Flexibility
- Muscular strength
- Muscular endurance

These components are linked to good health and reduced risk of *hypokinetic diseases*, which develop from lack of physical activity. Such diseases include cardiovascular disease, low back pain, musculoskeletal problems (relating to the interaction of muscles with bones and movement), obesity, diabetes, osteoprosis, and stress-related disorders.

Here are descriptions of the five components and some of the hypokinetic diseases related to each.

Cardiovascular Fitness

The ability of the heart, blood vessels, blood, and respiratory system to supply fuel and oxygen to the muscles and the ability of the muscles to sustain physical activity

Health concerns: cardiovascular disease, obesity

Body Composition

The relative percentage of muscle, fat, bone, and other tissues of the body—not just fat

Health concerns: cardiovascular disease, obesity, diabetes, musculoskeletal problems

Flexibility

The range of motion in a specific joint or area of the body, such as the shoulder or hip area

Health concern: musculoskeletal problems

Muscular Strength

The ability of the muscles to exert an external force, such as lift a heavy object

Health concern: musculoskeletal problems

Muscular Endurance

The ability of muscles to work repeatedly over a long period of time without fatigue

Health concerns: decreased work capacity and fatigue, musculoskeletal problems

Figure 7.2 Sample handout on the components of fitness.
*Adapted from Corbin, C. and Lindsey, R. (1991), *Concepts of Physical Fitness*. Dubuque, IA: Brown.

- Invite parents, school administrators, school board members, and other community leaders to observe testing.
- Present awards for supporting fitness at a special occasion in the community, such as a service club meeting.
- Place a bulletin-board display on health-related physical fitness in a public building such as a library.

Another idea is to create a physical education newsletter distributed several times a year. It could focus on the physical education program and have special sections devoted to fitness, including topics such as fitness testing, fitnessrelated knowledge, and specifics on those program activities designed to improve certain components of fitness.

Goal Setting*

Goal setting is a motivational strategy that can be used to increase exercise behavior (Locke, Shaw, Saari, & Latham, 1981). Whether used to encourage participation in exercise or improvement on future fitness test scores, goal setting is a valuable tool for children to learn. It teaches them how to plan and work to achieve their desires.

Setting Goals With Children

Your role in helping children set goals is twofold:

- To teach them the process of setting goals and planning how to reach them
- To guide them in selecting realistic but challenging goals

It is up to the child to decide what the goal or goals should be. At the beginning, you probably will have to give children a lot of suggestions and guidance in choosing goals, but you should need to do this less and less as they become more experienced. Follow these guidelines for setting goals (Gould, 1986):

1. Set goals together with students so that their interests are considered and they are committed to the goals.

2. Set goals that are based on students' past behavior or performance. If a student did 15 sit-ups on the pretest, then a goal might be to do 25 sit-ups on the posttest.

3. Set goals that are specific and measurable so students can tell if they have met or exceeded the goals. For instance, rather than setting a goal to "run faster" in the one-mile walk/run, state the goal as improving the time by 30 sec.

4. Set goals that are challenging but realistic. If a student did the mile run on the pretest in 12:45, a goal of running 5:15 on the posttest 8 weeks later is not realistic. To be motivational, goals must be achievable. Realistic goals take into account the time until the posttest, the current fitness level of the student, the student's age and sex, and the student's current level of physical activity.

5. Have students write down their goals. This helps students focus attention on the goals and keep them clear.

---

*Note. This section of chapter 7 is from "Goal Setting For Peak Performance" by D. Gould. In *Applied Sport Psychology: Personal Growth to Peak Performance* (2nd ed.) by J.M. Williams (Ed.), 1992, Mountain View, CA: Mayfield Publishing Co. Copyright © 1993 by Mayfield Publishing Company. Adapted by permission.

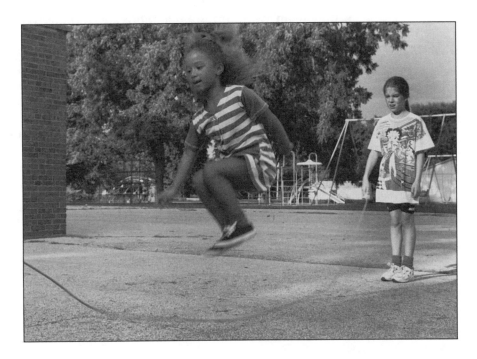

6. Help students understand how they can reach their goals. They need to know what types of activity to do to reach those goals and how to apply the FIT principle (frequency, intensity, time) to those activities.

7. Provide students with support and feedback about their progress toward their goals. Periodically ask students how they are doing. If you don't, students may think the goals aren't important to you and stop trying to achieve them.

8. Give students opportunities to assess their progress toward their goals by providing log sheets for recording exercise activity, doing periodic testing, or offering self-testing opportunities.

Also keep in mind that children should never set goals in comparison with one another. Goals should be set only against each child's own previous performance.

Consider these factors as you help each child develop specific goals:

- The child's sex and age. Males and females have some genetic differences that affect fitness performance. The maturational level of the student also will affect the types of fitness changes that can be expected.
- Time available for physical education. In your school system, how long is each class session? How many classes are there each week, and how many weeks are classes held?
- Time between pretesting and posttesting. Make sure that goals set for improving test scores are achievable within the time period between tests.
- The child's initial fitness level. Students starting at a low level of fitness should set goals of small increases in exercise behavior. Students who are already very fit may only be able to achieve small increments of improvement in their fitness.
- Exercise available outside of class. Physical Best (AAHPERD, 1989a) and FITNESSGRAM (Cooper Institute for Aerobics Research, 1992) use goal

setting in an award program to motivate students to participate in physical activities outside of physical education class. If it seems appropriate, and especially if there are attractive fitness options offered by the local park district, YMCA, or other youth-oriented organizations, you may want to encourage exercise outside of school.

Adjust your approach to teaching goal setting to the age of the students. Children as young as 6 can participate in goal setting, but such children will require more assistance from you in choosing realistic goals. They also should set no more than two goals, and those should be in the areas of most concern. More goals might become overwhelming to young children (See Figure 7.3 for sample goals for a younger student.)

Older children, with experience, can handle several goals at once (see Figure 7.4 for sample goals for an older student). Some fitness programs provide teachers and students computer assistance with goal setting (AAHPERD, 1989b; Dotson, 1989), particularly in identifying reasonable improvements that a child can achieve within a testing cycle based upon age and current fitness levels. These programs typically provide tracking mechanisms that also automatically

---

PROFILE: Female, 10 years of age

Does little physical activity outside of physical education class

---

Pretest results (20 weeks pre- to posttesting)

Muscular strength/muscular endurance

Upper body	Below criterion (0 pull-ups)
Abdominal	Below criterion (3 sit-ups)

Flexibility

Low back/hamstring	OK

Cardiovascular endurance

Mile-run test	Below criterion (12:10)

Body composition

Skinfold measures	Below criterion (38 mm skinfold = 30% fat)

We would choose to work on body composition first because this problem is probably affecting cardiovascular endurance and muscular strength/muscular endurance scores.

Posttest goal

Decrease sum of skinfolds (body composition) by 7 mm to a sum of skinfolds score of 31 mm.

Exercise goals

1. Participate in aerobic activity, such as riding bike, walking, or swimming, twice a week for 15 to 20 min, and walk once a week with a family member.
2. Eat fruits, vegetables, or other healthy foods as snacks when hungry between meals.

Figure 7.3 Sample of goal setting with a younger student.

indicate, after posttest results are entered, if a student has achieved the set goal. They may also provide feedback to the student about meeting the goal and what to do in the future to reach the goal. Such programs decrease the time you spend analyzing individual test results and can help if you are inexperienced at goal setting with children.

Which Goals: Improvement in Scores or Increased Participation?

Students can set goals for either increased participation in exercise or improvement in fitness testing scores. The means for reaching these two kinds of goals may be the same, but the child's ability to achieve them may differ. Which you encourage depends on what you want to emphasize in your program and on the children's present fitness levels.

Goal setting for improvement of test scores can increase the accuracy of tests that require children's maximal or near maximal efforts by motivating them to try their hardest. In addition it can help focus their minds on their own performance rather than how they stack up against classmates.

Goal setting for increased exercise participation is a way to develop good fitness habits for a lifetime. It encourages children to discover the joys of

---

PROFILE: Male, 16 years of age

Likes to play baseball and lift weights, no systematic stretching program

---

Pretest results (12 weeks pre- to posttesting)

Muscular strength/muscular endurance
    Upper body   OK
    Abdominal   OK
Flexibility
    Low back/hamstring   Below criterion (22 cm)
Cardiovascular endurance
    Mile-run test   Below criterion (8:10)
Body composition
    Skinfold measures   OK

Posttest goals

1. Increase score on sit-and-reach (flexibility) by 5 cm to a score of 27 cm.
2. Decrease mile-run time (cardiovascular endurance) by 45 sec to a time of 7:25.

Exercise goals

1. Participate in aerobic activity (running chosen as activity) 3 to 4 times a week for 20 to 30 minutes at target heart rate.
2. Complete daily stretching routine of static stretches for the low back/hamstring area (e.g., hamstring stretcher); hold each stretch for 10 to 15 sec and do each stretch 3 to 9 times.

Figure 7.4 Sample of goal setting for an older student.

movement and exercise and to try different types of exercise in order to find those they like.

If children are at high levels of fitness, it may be wiser to set goals for participation rather than improvement, because they are unlikely to improve by large amounts. Maintaining their already good fitness is more important. Children at low levels of fitness are more likely to make large gains in fitness scores, and if exercising is at first not attractive to them, perhaps improvement goals might be more motivating.

Awards

We can all remember the thrill of receiving a ribbon, medal, or certificate for achieving some special goal when we were children; we may also, however, remember what it felt like when others won them and we didn't. That is the paradox of awards. They can motivate, or they can discourage, in part based on how they are awarded. And they may not motivate as well as intrinsic motivators such as self-satisfaction or self-confidence. Whether you want to institute an award system and, if you do, how you want to structure that system depends on the philosophy of your program.

Awards and Motivation

Awards do not always increase motivation (Deci & Ryan, 1985); in fact, they can decrease it. How awards affect students is determined in part by why students believe the awards are given and whether they believe they can win them.

If students think they received an award because they did something well, then the award is likely to increase their motivation. If they believe, though, that they received the award for behaving a specific way the teacher wanted (the teacher is trying to control them), the award is likely to decrease their motivation. Students need to feel that their award reflects their competence.

In some fitness award systems only a few students can receive awards, based on their fitness scores. For instance, if only the top 15% can win awards, 85% of the students cannot. This often discourages the majority of the students. When students no longer believe that winning the award is an achievable goal, they will stop striving to reach the award standard. Unfortunately, the students who most need encouragement, those with low fitness levels, are the ones least likely to receive the encouragement of an award. In addition, such a rigid standard works against those who have reached adequate fitness but cannot excel because they are not genetically capable. If awards are based on the amount of improvement, a rigid standard may also work against those who are already at high levels of fitness.

Choosing the Award Criteria

If you decide that an award plan is appropriate for your program, you need to choose the award criteria. One of four criteria is usually chosen (Corbin, Whitehead, & Lovejoy, 1988):

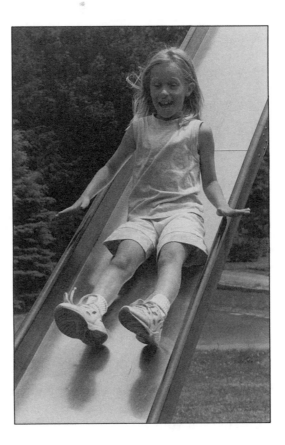

- *High-standard normative performance:* These awards are given to students who reach a specific score on a series of fitness tests in which the standards are based on how students compare with each other (PCPFS, 1985). For example, students would have to achieve scores in the 85th percentile of standards based on norms to receive an award.

- *Criterion-referenced standard performance:* Such awards go to students who reach or exceed a criterion-referenced standard.

- *Performance improvement:* Awards are granted on the basis of a certain amount of improvement on test scores.

- *Exercise behavior:* The awards go to students who complete a predetermined set of exercise behaviors over a given period of time.

Based on what we said previously about motivation and awards, the latter three are probably the most effective. You may want to have more than one award criterion in your program, since both good test performance and good exercise habits are desirable. We could even make the case that exercise behavior is more important, since a student who reaches the criterion standards today won't necessarily be fit for life.

Designing an Award System

If you choose to design your own award system, make sure that the criteria for the award reflect children's fitness competencies, including their ability to maintain good exercise behaviors. It's best to have different types of awards so all students' efforts can be recognized.

The item used as an award—a pin, patch, ribbon, or certificate—should be of little value in itself. Emphasize the child's accomplishment, not the award, which is only a symbol of that accomplishment.

Be sure to encourage those children who put forth a good effort but don't achieve the award criteria. If the only feedback given is the awards, those students who try but don't make it may become discouraged.

Program Evaluation

Up to now, we've focused on the use of testing results with individual children. However, results also can tell you something about your own success at teaching fitness. Test results can guide you in improving your physical education program.

Review your program after each round of testing. Begin by looking for patterns in the group test results. Are a majority of students falling below the criterion standards on cardiovascular endurance? Are there patterns when looking at test results by grade levels?

Then revise your program. Can you emphasize fitness components in which your students are weak? For cardiovascular endurance, include more activities that get students moving at moderate intensity for longer periods of time. For upper-body strength and endurance, choose games and exercises that require arm strength. If your program doesn't meet often enough for children to meet the fitness goals you think they can achieve, encourage students to participate in fitness activities outside of class (see the earlier "Setting Goals With Children").

Student Evaluation

The appropriate role of fitness test results in student evaluation, or grading, is difficult to determine. Ideally, if physical fitness objectives are part of the physical education curriculum, you would consider some aspects of fitness assessment in grading. But in reality, most programs today aren't able to dedicate enough time to fitness activities to make a great change in fitness scores. Unless your program has children in class 5 days a week for at least an hour, for 6 to 10 weeks, those children probably can't improve their scores from class work alone. And even in programs with this amount of time, some of the class period is taken up with motor skill development activities. If your classes don't allow children enough time to develop their fitness, it's unfair to grade them on improvement. This would be like using reading scores to determine students' grades but not allowing students to read in class.

One area of fitness that you could assess is children's cognitive knowledge about fitness. If you have developed objectives and taught lessons on fitness concepts, it seems fair to assess what children know about fitness and use it as a partial basis for grading.

We also think you should evaluate the affective component of your physical education program, although we don't recommend you use the results in grading. See what effect your program is having on children's attitudes and values in regard to fitness and physical activity.

Summary

- Share all fitness testing results with the students and explain them. Give each student a copy of the results written at the appropriate reading level.
- If possible, meet with children individually to discuss results. Younger children probably need more individual attention; older children may be better able to discuss the results as a group.
- Present an individual's results and their interpretation only to that individual. Word the feedback in a truthful but nonthreatening way. Be specific about each area of fitness tested.
- Tell students and assistants that all scores are confidential. Store scoring results in a secure place and, if necessary, use identification numbers rather than students' names on testing materials.
- Relate test results to fitness concepts, then ask students to develop their own exercise prescriptions.
- Before testing, inform parents about the nature of the testing and the feedback they and their child will receive. Stress that you have designed testing to be a positive experience and will keep all results confidential.
- After testing, send parents written information about their child's results, with explanatory material. Ask them to discuss the results with their child, and provide them with the child's fitness goal, if available.
- When possible, schedule conferences with parents to discuss test results. If conferences are not possible, offer parents a group presentation on physical fitness that includes distribution of students' test results.
- Try various means of educating the community about fitness year-round, including a physical education newsletter for parents.
- With students, set goals that are
  - developed together with students,
  - based on their own past performance,
  - specific and measurable,
  - challenging but realistic, and
  - written.
- Help students understand how to reach their goals, provide them with support and feedback, and offer them opportunities to assess their progress.
- Consider these factors when setting goals:
  - The child's sex and age
  - Time available for physical education
  - The child's initial fitness level
  - Opportunities available for exercise outside of class
  - Time between pretest and posttest
- Set one or two goals for younger children, several with older children.
- Goals for participation may be more appropriate for children at high levels of fitness; goals for test score improvement may be more appropriate for children at low levels of fitness.
- Awards can be motivating when students feel the award reflects their competency, not simply behavior that the teacher wants.
- Awards given only for high standards may discourage the majority of students.

- Awards usually are given for one of four criteria:
  - High-standard normative performance
  - Criterion-referenced standard performance
  - Performance improvement
  - Exercise behavior
- If you design your own award system, make sure the criteria reflect children's fitness competencies, and stress the accomplishment rather than the award. Awards for both exercise behavior and test score improvement are best. Encourage students who try, even if they don't achieve an award.
- Review your program after each round of testing and revise as necessary.
- Don't use test score improvement as a basis for grading unless sufficient class time is available for improving fitness. Cognitive knowledge of fitness is a valid basis for grading as long as you have taught the concepts being measured. Assess the affective results of your teaching, but don't use them as the basis for grades.

References

American Alliance for Health, Physical Education, Recreation and Dance. (1989a). *Physical Best: The AAHPERD guide to physical fitness education and assessment.* Reston, VA: Author.

American Alliance for Health, Physical Education, Recreation and Dance. (1989b). *Physical Best software.* Reston, VA: Author.

Cooper Institute for Aerobics Research. (1992). *FITNESSGRAM.* Dallas: Author.

Corbin, C.B., Whitehead, J.R., & Lovejoy, P.Y. (1988). Youth physical fitness awards. *Quest,* **40,** 200-218.

Deci, E.L., & Ryan, R.M. (1985). *Intrinsic motivation and self-determination in human behavior.* New York: Plenum Press.

Dotson, C.O. (1989). *Dino*Fit software system.* Burtonsville, MD: ARA/ Human Factors.

Gould, D. (1986). Goal setting for peak performance. In J.M. Williams (Ed.), *Applied sport psychology.* Champaign, IL: Human Kinetics.

Locke, E.A., Shaw, L.N., Saari, L.M., & Latham, G.P. (1981). Goal setting and task performance. *Psychological Bulletin,* **90,** 125-152.

Petray, C. (1990). Physical Best—PR tool for the elementary physical educator. *Journal of Physical Education, Recreation and Dance,* **62**(7), 23-26.

President's Council on Physical Fitness and Sports. (1985). *The Presidential Physical Fitness Award Program.* Washington, DC: Author.

CHAPTER 8

Fitness Education

Fitness testing is just one part of the total fitness education process. But how you view fitness, including fitness testing and its place in a physical education curriculum, depends on your personal philosophy of fitness. For example, do you consider fitness to be a stand-alone unit consisting of lesson plans for 6 to 8 weeks? Do you conduct fitness testing twice a year because it's a tradition to do so? Do you apply fitness and health concepts when teaching sport activities, motor skills, and games?

What Is Fitness Education?

Fitness education requires a much broader approach to fitness than that conventionally taught in schools. Instead of being confined to the typical multi-week unit, fitness education should be a long-term process that is integrated into all facets of your physical education curriculum. A well-designed program

- teaches basic health and fitness concepts,
- develops fitness and physical skills, and
- helps children acquire a positive attitude toward activities that contribute to overall fitness.

These three components reflect a proactive stance toward fitness in physical education. Your fitness education program should involve children in taking responsibility for their own fitness. It also should teach them to understand health-related concepts and appreciate the value of a healthy lifestyle—not just for today, but for a lifetime.

Implementation of a Fitness Education Program

How you implement your fitness education program depends on a variety of factors:

- School facilities
- Equipment
- School environment

- Students' ages
- Class size
- Maturity and experience levels of your students
- Length and frequency of classes
- Needs of your program
- Your knowledge of fitness and exercise physiology
- Your program philosophy and long-term goals for your students
- Administration/district philosophy and support for program
- Community programs

These factors will influence how you incorporate fitness education into your physical education curriculum. There are certain things, however, that most experts agree are important to establishing a developmentally appropriate fitness component in elementary physical education. Please keep the guidelines in the Fitness Checklist in mind as you develop and teach your fitness education program.

Fitness Checklist

Cautions

- Never use fitness activities as punishment.
- Never deny children fitness or skill education because of poor performance in other subjects.
- Don't overemphasize fitness testing.
- Don't underemphasize the importance of self-esteem to lifelong fitness. Avoid negative comments about poor performance.

Curriculum

- Create fitness programming that is appropriate for your students' developmental levels. Children are not miniature adults.
- Remember that fitness is for all children, not just athletically gifted ones. Design fitness activities to accommodate students of varying physical characteristics and levels of ability. Provide options for tasks to vary the level of difficulty.
- Teach fitness to complement the teaching of motor skills, movement concepts, dance, gymnastics, and games. Teaching children to move skillfully and to be physically fit are compatible goals.
- Make fitness fun!
- How you teach fitness will have a major impact on children's feelings about fitness and physical activity. Inspire competence and confidence in your students.
- Teach children fitness concepts for lifelong fitness. Fitness levels achieved during childhood will not last if students do not have the skills or motivation to continue to be active adults.
- Involve students in learning experiences that help them apply fitness information. Relate fitness concepts to everyday experiences.
- Use hands-on experience to provide students with challenges. Children learn best by hearing, seeing, and doing. Avoid lecturing as a typical approach to teaching fitness.

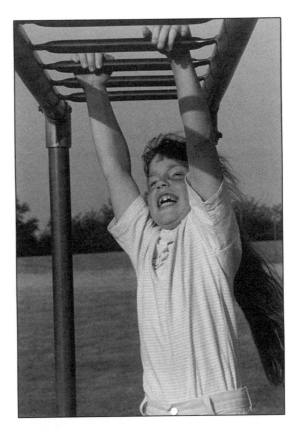

- Clarify goals and key points of your fitness lesson. Just because students do the activities doesn't mean they know why. Check for understanding.
- Remember that physical education specialists alone cannot make children fit. A cooperative effort is needed from parents, other teachers and school personnel, and the community.

Safety

- Use a general body, large muscle warm-up before vigorous and extensive exercise.
- Teach children the difference between initial fatigue and pain that may result in injury.
- Always make sure environmental conditions are safe for a fitness lesson.
- Be aware of harmful exercises. Research has found some traditional exercises—ones you may have learned in college—to be hazardous. Read current literature to doublecheck the safety of all your exercises.

This checklist represents just a few of the many factors that you need to consider when planning and developing a fitness education program. Undoubtedly you can think of many more that would apply to your situation.

Annotated List of Resources

If you would like more information to help you develop your fitness education program, please consider the list of resources in this section.

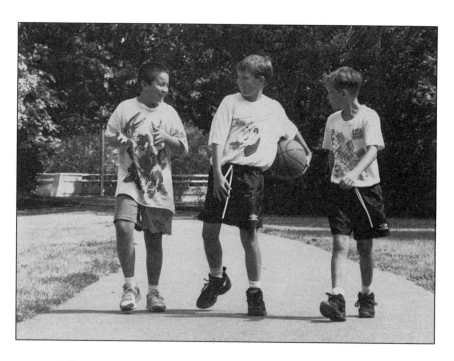

Suggested Readings

Cooper, K. (1991). *Kid's fitness*. New York: Bantam.

> A book for parents, teachers, and coaches on the topic of exercise and nutrition for children and adolescents. Information includes child development, motivational strategies, exercise programs, and nutritional advice to promote children's physical fitness and self-esteem.

Corbin, C.B. (1987). Physical fitness in the K-12 curriculum: Some defensible solutions to perennial problems. *Journal of Physical Education, Recreation and Dance*, **58**(7), 49-54.

> Explains the importance of teaching higher order objectives. Describes problems associated with teaching fitness in school situations and offers constructive solutions.

Corbin, C.B., & Lindsey, R. (1991). *Concepts of physical fitness with laboratories* (7th ed). Dubuque, IA: Brown.

> Textbook designed for an introductory physical fitness and exercise class at the college level. Excellent detailed fitness information.

Corbin, C.B., & Lindsey, R. (1990). *Fitness for life* (3rd ed.). Glenview, IL: Scott, Foresman.

> Textbook for junior-high and high-school students.

Corbin, C.B., & Pangrazi, R.P. (1989). *Teaching strategies for improving youth fitness*. Dallas: Cooper Institute for Aerobics Research.

> Fitness information and learning activities for elementary through high-school students.

Foster, E.R., Hartinger, K., & Smith, K.A. (1992). *Fitness fun*. Champaign, IL: Human Kinetics.

> Book of 85 field-tested fitness games and activities for children from K to 8. Codes games and activities to show which fitness components are emphasized. Includes warm-up activities, short activities, and longer main activities.

Glover, D.R., & Midura, D.W. (1992). *Team building through physical challenges.* Champaign, IL: Human Kinetics.

A set of 22 Outward Bound-type physical challenge tasks to help students in upper elementary through high school build interpersonal skills as well as motor skills. Includes cards that explain each challenge to students.

Graham, G. (1992). *Teaching children physical education: Becoming a master teacher.* Champaign, IL: Human Kinetics.

Text for the Pedagogy Course of the American Master Teacher Program for Children's Physical Education. Focuses on successful teaching skills and techniques used by master teachers.

Gustafson, M.A., Wolfe, S.K., & King, C.L. (1991). *Great games for young people.* Champaign, IL: Human Kinetics.

Book of 69 field-tested games for upper-elementary to senior-high students. Complete description and suggested modifications for each game.

Hopple, C. (1995). *Teaching for outcomes in elementary physical education.* Champaign, IL: Human Kinetics.

A guide to outcomes-based education, part of the American Master Teacher Program. Describes how to use outcomes for curriculum planning and how to define authentic performance and portfolio tasks for assessment. Provides relevant cues and activities for 23 basic PE skills and concepts.

Hopple, C. (Ed.) *Teaching Elementary Physical Education (TEPE).*

A bimonthly newsletter for elementary physical educators. Available from Child Health Division, Human Kinetics Publishers.

McSwegin, P.J., Pemberton, C., Petray, C., Blazer, S., Lavay, B., & Leads, M. (1989). Fitting in fitness. *Journal of Physical Education, Recreation and Dance,* **60**(1), 30-45.

A special feature with several articles on planning a fitness curriculum, fitness testing, and helping students set goals and stay motivated.

Morris, G.S.D., & Stiehl, J. (1989). *Changing kids' games.* Champaign, IL: Human Kinetics.

Presents a model for selecting, planning, modifying, presenting, and evaluating movement games for children in K to 8. Helps instructors add new twists to traditional games.

Petray, C.K., & Blaer, S.L. (1991). *Health related physical fitness: Concepts and activities for elementary school children* (3rd ed.). Edina, MN: Bellwether Press.

Textbook for teachers includes comprehensive information about health-related fitness with practical activities for children.

Pica, R., & Gardzina, R. (1991). *Early elementary children moving and learning.* Champaign, IL: Human Kinetics.

A 5-cassette set with a 3-ring notebook contains this complete movement program for K to 3 children. Includes 40 developmentally appropriate lesson plans and 200 movement activities, with music written especially for the program.

Pica, R. (1991). *Special themes for moving & learning.* Champaign, IL: Human Kinetics.

Movement activities for children 4 to 8 covering 38 themes such as holidays, animals, and seasons.

Ratliffe, T., & Ratliffe, L. (1994). *Teaching children fitness: Becoming a master teacher.* Champaign, IL: Human Kinetics.

Text from the American Master Teacher Program on how to develop a

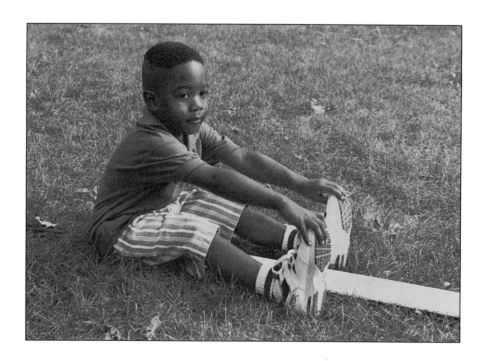

developmentally appropriate and sound physical education curriculum. Reflects the views of children's physical education expressed in NASPE's *Physically Educated Person* and COPEC's *Appropriate Physical Education for Children* documents.

Rowland, T.W. (1990). *Exercise and children's health*. Champaign, IL: Human Kinetics.

Comprehensive reference book describes the changes in physiological responses to exercise that occur as children grow, summarizes the evidence linking exercise to health in children, and provides guidelines for counseling children into more active lifestyles.

Simons-Morton, B.G., O'Hara, N.M., Simons-Morton, D.G., & Parcel, G.S. (1987). Children and fitness: A public health perspective. *Research Quarterly for Exercise and Sport*, **58**, (4), 295-302.

Summarizes the following issues regarding children's physical fitness: the current status of children's cardiorespiratory fitness; the effects of childhood training programs on the fitness of children and of training programs on the fitness of children and adults; the extent of children's participation in moderate to vigorous physical activity; and the potential for, and role of, physical education in promoting children's lifelong fitness and health.

Solis, K.M., & Burdis, B. (1991). *The jump rope primer*. Champaign, IL: Human Kinetics.

A complete jump rope program, with illustrated skills from simple to complex and an eight-lesson unit that takes students from the basic two-foot jump to Double Dutch routines. Stretching routines, jump rope games, and other background information included.

Solis, K.M., & Budris, B. (1991). *The jump rope primer video*. Champaign, IL: Human Kinetics.

A 32-min videotape. Video that accompanies *The Jump Rope Primer*. Demonstrates all the jump rope techniques in the manual.

Stillwell, J.L. (1987). *Making and using creative play equipment*. Champaign, IL: Human Kinetics.

Practical information on how to construct equipment for activities that develop locomotor, manipulative, and perceptual-motor skills and for organizing activities. Includes suggested activities.

Strand, B.N., & Wilson, R. (1993). *Assessing sport skills*. Champaign, IL: Human Kinetics.

A comprehensive guide to 379 tests in 29 sports and activities. Includes background information on how to choose the right test and proper testing procedures. Tables and diagrams illustrate how to administer each test.

Thomas, J.R., Lee, A.M., & Thomas, K.T. (1988). *Physical education for children: Concepts into practice*. Champaign, IL: Human Kinetics.

A text on how to teach quality physical education classes. Covers children's physical development, curriculum planning and class organization, and evaluating and improving teaching.

Thomas, J.R., Lee, A.M., & Thomas, K.T. (1989). *Physical education for children: Daily lesson plans*. Champaign, IL: Human Kinetics.

Companion piece to *Concepts Into Practice* includes 376 lesson plans for children K to 8. Four activity areas are covered: fitness, games and sports, rhythmic activities, and gymnastics.

Whitehead, J.R. (1992). A selected, annotated bibliography for fitness educators. *Journal of Physical Education, Recreation and Dance*, **63**(5), 53-64.

Comprehensive annotated bibliography on the topic of youth fitness provides excellent references for fitness educators.

Wnek, B. (1992). *Holiday games and activities*. Champaign, IL: Human Kinetics.

A compilation of physical fitness activities, skills, games, rhythm and dance activities, and bulletin-board ideas for each of eight seasons and holidays. Activities are for children K to 6.

Additional Resources

American Cancer Society (listed in white pages of telephone book). Instructional package containing lesson plans and videotapes.

American Heart Association (listed in white pages of telephone book). Program Packages contain teacher's guide, posters, videotapes, and learning experiences.

Heart Treasure Chest (3-5 years)
Getting to Know Your Heart (lower elementary)
Getting to Know Your Heart (upper elementary)
Fit to Achieve Elementary Cardiovascular Education Program Physical Education Program

Division of Curriculum & Instruction
University of North Florida
4567 St. Johns Bluff Rd.
Jacksonville, FL 32224

For two 13-min videotaped programs and printed materials send a check for $20. Make check payable to Division of Curriculum & Instruction. Cardiovascular educational fitness materials include two instructional videos, student assignments and worksheets, a teacher's guide, and a parent's guide.

Creative Walking Incorporated
P.O. Box 50296
Clayton, MD 63105

Information is provided to help you design a walking wellness curriculum for children. A workbook for elementary-aged students helps them learn about and practice fitness activities.

Healthy Growing Up
McDonald's Education Resource Center
P.O. Box 8002
St. Charles, IL 60174-8002
800-627-7646

Lessons are designed to encourage children (Grades K-3) to adopt lifelong habits of good nutrition, exercise, and positive self-esteem.

Kimbo Educational Records
P.O. Box 477
Long Branch, NJ 07740-0477
800-631-2187

Aerobic exercise videotapes for children.

Slim Goodbody VideoKits
AV Instructional Services
Agency for Instructional Technology
Box A
Bloomington, Indiana 47402-9973

THE INSIDE STORY: Ten 15-min video programs present the exciting story of the human body, with working models of organs and body systems.

ALL FIT: Fifteen 15-min video programs feature vigorous, structured exercises easily done in the classroom, each highlighting a fitness topic and a major muscle group.

WELL, WELL, WELL: This series of fifteen 15-min video programs shows how even young children can take an active part in protecting and maintaining their good health. The emphasis is on wellness, safety, nutrition, exercise, and handling feelings in a healthy way.

Sources for Fitness Testing Equipment

Skinfold Calipers/Adipometers

Fat-O-Meter

> Health Education Services Corp.
> 7N015 York Rd.
> Bensenville, IL 60106

Slim Guide

> Creative Health Products
> 9135 General Circle
> Plymouth, MI 48170

Physique Meter

> Dr. H. Co
> P.O. Box 266
> Chesterfield, MO 63017

Harpenden

> Quinton Instrument Co.
> 2121 Terry Ave.
> Seattle, WA 98121

Lange

> J.A. Preston Corp.
> 71 Fifth Ave.
> New York, NY 10013

> Cambridge Scentific Industries
> P.O. Box 265
> Cambridge, MD 21613
> 800-638-9566

Adipometer

Ross Laboratories
Educational Services Department
625 Cleveland Ave.
Columbus, OH 43216
614-624-7900

PACER Music Tape and Wall Chart

The Prudential FITNESSGRAM
Cooper Institute for Aerobics Research
12330 Preston Rd.
Dallas, TX 75230

Equipment for Back Saver Sit-and-Reach

1. Using any sturdy wood or comparable material (3/4-in. plywood seems to work well), cut the following pieces:
   2 pieces, 12 in. by 12 in.
   2 pieces, 12 in. by 10-1/2 in.
   1 piece, 12 in. by 22 in.

2. Cut pieces that are 10 in. by 4 in. from each side of one end of the 12 in. by 22 in. piece to make the top of the box (see diagram). Beginning at the small end, make marks on the piece each inch up to 12 in.

3. Construct a box from the remaining four pieces using nails, screws, or wood glue. Attach the top of the box. It is crucial that the 9-in. mark be exactly in line with the vertical plane against which the subject's feet will be placed. The 0-in. mark is at the end that will be nearest the subject.

4. Cover the apparatus with polyurethane sealer or shellac.

Alternate Flexibility Testing Apparatus

1. Find a sturdy cardboard box at least 12 in. tall. Turn the box so that the bottom is up. Tape a yardstick to the bottom. The yardstick must be placed so that the 9-in. mark is exactly in line with the vertical plane against which the subject's feet will be placed and the 0-in. end is nearer the subject.

2. Find a bench that is about 12 in. wide. Turn the bench on its side. Tape a yardstick to the bench so that the 9-in. mark is exactly in line with the

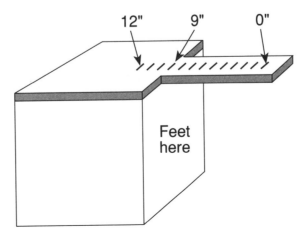

vertical plane against which the subject's feet will be placed and the 0-in. end is nearer the subject.

Equipment for Modified Pull-Up

Items needed

1 3/4-in. plywood, 24 in. by 39 in. dimensions, for support platform
2 2 in. by 8 in. by 24 in. pieces for base of uprights
2 2 in. by 4 in. by 48 in. pieces for uprights
1 1-1/8 in. steel pipe for chinning bar
1 1-1/4 in. dowel for top support
24 3/8-in. dowel pieces cut 3-1/2 in. long
Nails, wood screws, and wood glue for construction

1. Beginning 2-1/2-in. from the top end of the 2 by 4 by 48 pieces drill one hole through the 2-in. width for the 1-1/4 in. dowel support rod (see diagram a).
2. Drill eleven 1-1/8 in. holes below the first hole, measuring 2-1/2 in. between the centers of these holes.
3. Beginning 3-3/4 in. from the top of these upright pieces, drill 12 3/8-in. holes into the 4-in. width. Center these holes between the holes for the steel rod (see diagram b).
4. Assemble the pieces and finish with polyurethane or shellac.

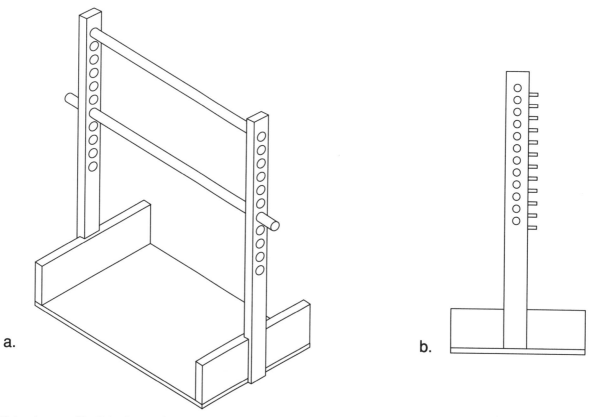

a.   b.

APPENDIX C

NCYFS I Norms (ages 10-18)

Table A.1   NCYFS I Norms by Age for the One-Mile Walk/Run—Boys
(in Minutes:Seconds)

	Age								
Percentile	10	11	12	13	14	15	16	17	18
99	6:55	6:21	6:21	5:59	5:43	5:40	5:31	5:14	5:33
90	8:13	7:25	7:13	6:48	6:27	6:23	6:13	6:08	6:10
80	8:35	7:52	7:41	7:07	6:58	6:43	6:31	6:31	6:33
75	8:48	8:02	7:53	7:14	7:08	6:52	6:39	6:40	6:42
70	9:02	8:12	8:03	7:24	7:18	7:00	6:50	6:46	6:57
60	9:26	8:38	8:23	7:46	7:34	7:13	7:07	7:10	7:15
50	9:52	9:03	8:48	8:04	7:51	7:30	7:27	7:31	7:35
40	10:15	9:25	9:17	8:26	8:14	7:50	7:48	7:59	7:53
30	10:44	10:17	9:57	8:54	8:46	8:18	8:04	8:24	8:12
25	11:00	10:32	10:13	9:06	9:10	8:30	8:18	8:37	8:34
20	11:25	10:55	10:38	9:20	9:28	8:50	8:34	8:55	9:10
10	12:27	12:07	11:48	10:38	10:34	10:13	9:36	10:43	10:50

Table A.2   NCYFS I Norms by Age for the One-Mile Walk/Run—Girls (in Minutes:Seconds)

Percentile	Age								
	10	11	12	13	14	15	16	17	18
99	7:55	7:14	7:20	7:08	7:01	6:59	7:03	6:52	6:58
90	9:09	8:45	8:34	8:27	8:11	8:23	8:28	8:20	8:22
80	9:56	9:35	9:30	9:13	8:49	9:04	9:06	9:10	9:27
75	10:09	9:56	9:52	9:30	9:16	9:28	9:25	9:26	9:31
70	10:27	10:10	10:05	9:48	9:31	9:49	9:41	9:41	9:36
60	10:51	10:35	10:32	10:22	10:04	10:20	10:15	10:16	10:08
50	11:14	11:15	10:58	10:52	10:32	10:46	10:34	10:34	10:51
40	11:54	11:46	11:26	11:22	10:58	11:20	11:08	10:59	11:27
30	12:27	12:33	12:03	11:55	11:35	11:53	11:49	11:43	11:58
25	12:52	12:54	12:33	12:17	11:49	12:18	12:10	12:03	12:14
20	13:12	13:17	12:53	12:43	12:10	12:48	12:32	12:30	12:37
10	14:20	14:35	14:07	13:45	13:13	14:07	13:42	13:46	15:18

Table A.3   NCYFS I Norms by Age for the Timed Bent-Knee Sit-Ups—Boys (Number in 60 Seconds)

Percentile	Age								
	10	11	12	13	14	15	16	17	18
99	60	60	61	62	64	65	65	68	67
90	47	48	50	52	52	53	55	56	54
80	43	43	46	48	49	50	51	51	50
75	40	41	44	46	47	48	49	50	50
70	38	40	43	45	45	46	48	49	48
60	36	38	40	41	43	44	45	46	44
50	34	36	38	40	41	42	43	43	43
40	32	34	35	37	39	40	41	41	40
30	30	31	33	34	37	37	39	39	38
25	28	30	32	32	35	36	38	37	36
20	26	28	30	31	34	35	36	35	35
10	22	22	25	28	30	31	32	31	31

Table A.4   NCYFS I Norms by Age for the Timed Bent-Knee Sit-Ups—Girls (Number in 60 Seconds)

Percentile	Age								
	10	11	12	13	14	15	16	17	18
99	50	53	66	58	57	56	59	60	65
90	43	42	46	46	47	45	49	47	47
80	39	39	41	41	42	42	42	41	42
75	37	37	40	40	41	40	40	40	40
70	36	36	39	39	40	39	39	39	40
60	33	34	36	35	37	36	37	37	38
50	31	32	33	33	35	35	35	36	35
40	30	30	31	31	32	32	33	33	33
30	27	28	30	28	30	30	30	31	30
25	25	26	28	27	29	30	30	30	30
20	24	24	27	25	27	28	28	29	28
10	20	20	21	21	23	24	23	24	24

Table A.5   NCYFS I Norms by Age for the Sit-and-Reach—Boys (in Inches)

Percentile	Age								
	10	11	12	13	14	15	16	17	18
99	18.0	18.5	18.5	19.5	20.0	21.5	22.0	21.5	22.0
90	16.0	16.5	16.0	16.5	17.5	18.0	19.0	19.5	19.5
80	15.0	15.5	15.0	15.0	16.0	17.0	18.0	18.0	18.0
75	14.5	15.0	15.0	15.0	15.5	16.5	17.0	17.5	17.5
70	14.5	14.5	14.5	14.5	15.0	16.0	17.0	17.0	17.0
60	14.0	14.0	13.5	13.5	14.0	15.0	16.0	16.0	16.0
50	13.5	13.0	13.0	13.0	13.5	14.0	15.0	15.5	15.0
40	12.5	12.5	12.0	12.5	13.0	13.5	14.0	14.5	14.5
30	12.0	12.0	11.5	12.0	12.0	12.5	13.5	13.5	13.5
25	11.5	11.5	11.0	11.0	11.0	12.0	13.0	13.0	13.0
20	11.0	11.0	10.5	10.5	11.0	11.5	12.0	12.5	12.5
10	10.0	9.5	8.5	9.0	9.0	9.5	10.0	10.5	10.0

Note: The 1980 AAHPERD norms used a "0" point of 23 cm, but NCYFS used 12 in. To adjust the "0" point and to change inches to centimeters, use the following formula: Score in centimeters = (Score in inches × 2.54) − 7.48. From the National Children and Youth Fitness Study.

Table A.6   NCYFS I Norms by Age for the Sit-and-Reach—Girls (in Inches)

Percentile	Age								
	10	11	12	13	14	15	16	17	18
99	20.5	20.5	21.0	22.0	22.0	23.0	23.0	23.0	22.5
90	17.5	18.0	19.0	20.0	19.5	20.0	20.5	20.5	20.5
80	16.5	17.0	18.0	19.0	19.0	19.0	19.5	19.5	19.5
75	16.5	16.5	17.0	18.0	18.5	19.0	19.0	19.0	19.0
70	16.0	16.5	17.0	17.5	18.0	18.5	19.0	19.0	18.5
60	15.0	15.5	16.0	17.0	17.5	18.0	18.0	18.0	18.0
50	14.5	15.0	15.5	16.0	17.0	17.0	17.5	18.0	17.5
40	14.0	14.0	15.0	15.5	16.0	17.0	17.0	17.0	17.0
30	13.0	13.5	14.5	14.5	15.0	16.0	16.5	16.0	16.0
25	13.0	13.0	14.0	14.0	15.0	15.5	16.0	15.5	15.5
20	12.0	13.0	13.5	13.5	14.0	15.0	15.5	15.0	15.0
10	10.5	11.5	12.0	12.0	12.5	13.5	14.0	13.5	13.0

Note: The 1980 AAHPERD norms used a "0" point of 23 cm, but NCYFS used 12 in. To adjust the "0" point and to change inches to centimeters, use the following formula: Score in centimeters = (Score in inches × 2.54) − 7.48. From the National Children and Youth Fitness Study.

Table A.7   NCYFS I Norms by Age for the Triceps Skinfold—Boys (in Millimeters)

Percentile	Age								
	10	11	12	13	14	15	16	17	18
99	5	4	4	4	4	4	4	4	4
90	7	7	6	6	5	5	5	5	5
80	8	7	8	7	6	6	6	6	6
75	8	8	8	7	7	7	6	6	6
70	9	9	9	8	7	7	7	7	7
60	10	10	10	9	8	8	7	7	8
50	11	11	11	10	9	9	8	8	8
40	13	12	12	11	10	10	9	9	10
30	14	14	14	13	11	11	11	11	11
25	15	15	15	14	12	12	11	12	12
20	16	16	17	15	13	13	12	13	13
10	20	20	21	20	18	18	16	15	16

Table A.8 NCYFS I Norms by Age for the Triceps Skinfold—Girls (in Millimeters)

Percentile	Age								
	10	11	12	13	14	15	16	17	18
99	5	6	6	6	6	7	7	8	7
90	7	8	9	9	9	10	10	11	10
80	9	9	10	10	11	12	12	12	12
75	10	10	10	11	12	13	12	13	13
70	10	10	11	11	12	13	13	14	13
60	11	12	12	13	14	15	14	15	14
50	12	13	13	14	15	16	15	17	15
40	14	15	14	15	16	17	17	18	17
30	15	16	16	17	18	19	18	20	19
25	16	17	17	18	19	20	19	21	20
20	17	19	18	20	20	21	20	21	21
10	21	23	22	24	23	25	24	24	23

Table A.9 NCYFS I Norms by Age for the Triceps and Subscapular Skinfolds—Boys (in Millimeters)

Percentile	Age								
	10	11	12	13	14	15	16	17	18
99	9	9	9	9	9	10	10	10	11
90	12	12	12	11	12	12	12	13	13
80	13	13	13	13	13	13	13	14	14
75	14	14	14	13	13	14	14	14	15
70	15	15	15	14	14	14	14	15	15
60	16	16	16	15	15	15	15	16	17
50	17	18	17	17	17	17	17	17	18
40	20	20	20	19	18	18	18	19	19
30	22	23	22	21	21	20	20	21	22
25	24	25	24	23	22	22	22	22	24
20	25	26	28	25	25	24	23	24	25
10	35	36	38	34	33	32	30	30	30

Table A.10   NCYFS I Norms by Age for the Triceps and Subscapular Skinfolds—
Girls (in Millimeters)

Percentile	Age								
	10	11	12	13	14	15	16	17	18
99	10	11	11	12	12	13	13	16	14
90	13	14	15	15	17	19	19	20	19
80	15	16	17	18	19	21	21	22	21
75	16	17	18	19	20	23	22	23	22
70	17	18	18	20	21	24	23	24	23
60	18	19	21	22	24	26	24	26	25
50	20	21	22	24	26	28	26	28	27
40	22	24	24	26	28	30	28	31	28
30	25	28	27	29	31	33	32	34	32
25	27	30	29	31	33	34	33	36	34
20	29	33	31	34	35	37	35	37	36
10	36	40	40	43	40	43	42	42	42

Table A.11   NCYFS I Norms by Age for the Chin-up—Boys (Number Completed)

Percentile	Age								
	10	11	12	13	14	15	16	17	18
99	13	12	13	17	18	18	20	20	21
90	8	8	8	10	12	14	14	15	16
80	5	5	6	8	9	11	12	13	14
75	4	5	5	7	8	10	12	12	13
70	4	4	5	7	8	10	11	12	12
60	2	3	4	5	6	8	10	10	11
50	1	2	3	4	5	7	9	9	10
40	1	1	2	3	4	6	8	8	9
30	0	0	1	1	3	5	6	6	7
25	0	0	0	1	2	4	6	5	6
20	0	0	0	0	1	3	5	4	5
10	0	0	0	0	0	1	2	2	3

Table A.12   NCYFS I Norms by Age for the Chin-up—Girls (Number Completed)

Percentile	Age								
	10	11	12	13	14	15	16	17	18
99	8	8	8	5	8	6	8	7	6
90	3	3	2	2	2	2	2	2	2
80	2	1	1	1	1	1	1	1	1
75	1	1	1	1	1	1	1	1	1
70	1	1	1	0	1	1	1	1	1
60	0	0	0	0	0	0	0	0	0
50	0	0	0	0	0	0	0	0	0
40	0	0	0	0	0	0	0	0	0
30	0	0	0	0	0	0	0	0	0
25	0	0	0	0	0	0	0	0	0
20	0	0	0	0	0	0	0	0	0
10	0	0	0	0	0	0	0	0	0

NCYFS II Norms (ages 6-9)

Table A.13   NCYFS II Norms by Age for the Distance Walk/Run (in Minutes:Seconds)

	Age							
	Boys				Girls			
	Half-mile		Mile		Half-mile		Mile	
Percentile	6	7	8	9	6	7	8	9
99	3:53	3:34	7:42	7:31	4:05	4:03	8:18	8:06
95	4:15	3:56	8:18	7:54	4:29	4:18	9:14	8:41
90	4:27	4:11	8:46	8:10	4:46	4:32	9:39	9:08
85	4:35	4:22	9:02	8:33	4:57	4:38	9:55	9:26
80	4:45	4:28	9:19	8:48	5:07	4:46	10:08	9:40
75	4:52	4:33	9:29	9:00	5:13	4:54	10:23	9:50
70	4:59	4:40	9:40	9:13	5:20	5:00	10:35	10:15
65	5:04	4:46	9:52	9:29	5:25	5:06	10:46	10:31
60	5:10	4:50	10:04	9:44	5:31	5:11	10:59	10:41
55	5:17	4:54	10:16	9:58	5:39	5:18	11:14	10:56
50	5:23	5:00	10:39	10:10	5:44	5:25	11:32	11:13
45	5:28	5:05	11:00	10:27	5:49	5:32	11:46	11:30
40	5:33	5:11	11:14	10:41	5:55	5:39	12:03	11:46
35	5:41	5:17	11:30	10:59	6:00	5:46	12:14	12:09
30	5:50	5:28	11:51	11:16	6:07	5:55	12:37	12:26
25	5:58	5:35	12:14	11:44	6:14	6:01	12:59	12:45
20	6:09	5:46	12:39	12:02	6:27	6:10	13:26	13:13
15	6:21	6:06	13:16	12:46	6:39	6:20	14:18	13:44
10	6:40	6:20	14:05	13:37	6:51	6:38	14:48	14:31
5	7:15	6:50	15:24	15:15	7:16	7:09	16:35	15:40

This table is reprinted with permission from the JOPERD (Journal of Physical Education, Recreation & Dance) Nov-Dec, 1987, p. 70. JOPERD is a publication of the American Alliance for Health, Physical Education, Recreation and Dance, 1900 Association Drive, Reston, VA 22091-1599.

Table A.14   NCYFS II Norms by Age for the Timed Bent-Knee Sit-Ups (Number in 60 Seconds)

	Age							
	Boys				Girls			
Percentile	6	7	8	9	6	7	8	9
99	36	42	43	48	36	40	44	43
95	31	35	38	42	31	35	37	39
90	28	32	35	39	28	33	34	36
85	26	30	33	36	26	30	32	34
80	25	29	32	35	24	28	30	32
75	24	28	30	33	23	27	29	31
70	22	27	29	32	22	26	28	30
65	21	26	28	31	21	24	27	29
60	20	25	27	30	20	23	26	28
55	19	24	26	29	19	22	25	26
50	19	23	26	28	18	21	25	26
45	18	22	25	27	17	21	24	25
40	17	21	24	26	17	20	23	24
35	16	20	23	25	16	19	21	23
30	15	19	21	24	15	17	20	22
25	14	18	20	23	14	16	19	21
20	12	16	19	22	12	15	17	19
15	11	14	17	19	10	13	16	17
10	9	12	15	16	6	11	13	15
5	4	7	11	13	1	7	9	10

This table is reprinted with permission from the JOPERD (Journal of Physical Education, Recreation & Dance), Nov-Dec, 1987, p. 70. JOPERD is a publication of the American Alliance for Health, Physical Education, Recreation and Dance, 1900 Association Drive, Reston, VA 22091-1599.

Table A.15   NCYFS II Norms by Age for the Sit-and-Reach (in Inches)

| | Age | | | | | | | |
| | Boys | | | | Girls | | | |
Percentile	6	7	8	9	6	7	8	9
99	17.5	18.0	18.0	17.5	18.5	18.0	19.0	19.0
95	16.5	16.5	16.5	16.0	17.5	17.5	17.5	18.0
90	16.0	16.0	16.0	15.5	16.5	17.0	17.0	17.0
85	15.5	16.0	15.5	15.0	16.0	16.5	16.5	16.5
80	15.0	15.5	15.0	14.5	16.0	16.0	16.0	16.0
75	15.0	15.0	14.5	14.5	15.5	16.0	16.0	16.0
70	14.5	14.5	14.5	14.0	15.0	15.5	15.5	15.5
65	14.0	14.0	14.0	14.0	15.0	15.0	15.0	15.0
60	14.0	14.0	14.0	13.5	15.0	15.0	15.0	15.0
55	13.5	13.5	13.5	13.0	14.5	15.0	14.5	14.5
50	13.5	13.5	13.5	13.0	14.0	14.5	14.0	14.0
45	13.0	13.0	13.0	12.5	14.0	14.5	14.0	14.0
40	12.5	12.5	12.5	12.0	14.0	14.0	13.5	14.0
35	12.5	12.5	12.5	12.0	13.5	14.0	13.5	13.5
30	12.0	12.0	12.0	11.5	13.0	13.5	13.0	13.0
25	12.0	11.5	11.5	11.0	12.5	13.0	12.5	12.5
20	11.5	11.5	11.0	10.5	12.0	12.5	12.0	12.0
15	11.0	11.0	10.5	10.0	12.0	12.0	11.5	11.5
10	10.5	10.0	9.5	9.5	11.5	11.5	11.0	11.0
5	10.0	9.0	8.5	8.0	10.5	10.5	10.5	9.0

Note: The NCYFS set the ''0'' point at 12 in., whereas the 1980 AAHPERD norms employed a ''0'' point of 23 cm. To translate the NCYFS inches into centimeters and to adjust the ''0'' point to 23 cm, the following formula may be applied to the NCYFS norms: Score in cm = (Score in inches × 2.54) − 7.48.

This table is reprinted with permission from the JOPERD (Journal of Physical Education, Recreation & Dance), Nov-Dec, 1987, p. 68. JOPERD is a publication of the American Alliance for Health, Physical Education, Recreation and Dance, 1900 Association Drive, Reston, VA 22091-1599.

Table A.16   NCYFS II Norms by Age for the Triceps Skinfold (in Millimeters)

	Age							
	Boys				Girls			
Percentile	6	7	8	9	6	7	8	9
99	5	5	5	5	5	6	6	6
95	6	5	6	6	7	7	7	7
90	6	6	6	6	8	7	8	8
85	7	7	7	7	8	8	8	9
80	7	7	7	7	9	8	9	10
75	7	7	7	8	9	9	9	10
70	7	7	8	8	9	9	10	11
65	8	8	8	9	10	10	10	11
60	8	8	8	10	10	10	11	12
55	8	8	9	10	11	11	12	12
50	8	9	9	10	11	11	12	13
45	9	9	10	11	12	12	13	14
40	9	10	10	12	12	12	14	14
35	10	10	11	13	13	13	15	15
30	10	11	12	14	13	13	16	16
25	10	11	13	15	14	14	17	18
20	11	12	14	16	14	15	18	19
15	12	14	15	18	15	17	19	21
10	13	16	19	21	17	19	21	22
5	16	20	23	23	20	22	25	25

This table is reprinted with permission from the JOPERD (Journal of Physical Education, Recreation & Dance), Nov-Dec, 1987, p. 66. JOPERD is a publication of the American Alliance for Health, Physical Education, Recreation and Dance, 1900 Association Drive, Reston, VA 22091-1599.

Table A.17　NCYFS II Norms by Age for the Subscapular Skinfold (in Millimeters)

	Age							
	Boys				Girls			
Percentile	6	7	8	9	6	7	8	9
99	4	4	4	4	4	4	4	4
95	4	4	4	4	4	4	5	5
90	4	4	4	5	5	5	5	5
85	4	5	5	5	5	5	5	5
80	5	5	5	5	5	5	5	6
75	5	5	5	5	5	5	6	6
70	5	5	5	5	5	5	6	6
65	5	5	5	6	6	6	6	6
60	5	5	5	6	6	6	6	7
55	5	5	6	6	6	6	6	7
50	5	5	6	6	6	6	7	7
45	5	6	6	7	6	7	7	8
40	6	6	6	7	7	7	8	9
35	6	6	6	7	7	7	8	9
30	6	6	7	8	7	8	9	10
25	6	7	7	9	8	9	10	12
20	7	7	8	10	8	10	12	15
15	7	8	10	12	10	11	15	17
10	8	10	14	15	12	13	17	21
5	12	16	19	20	16	19	21	25

This table is reprinted with permission from the JOPERD (Journal of Physical Education, Recreation & Dance), Nov-Dec, 1987, p. 67. JOPERD is a publication of the American Alliance for Health, Physical Education, Recreation and Dance, 1900 Association Drive, Reston, VA 22091-1599.

Table A.18   NCYFS II Norms by Age for the Medial Calf Skinfold (in Millimeters)

	Age							
	Boys				Girls			
Percentile	6	7	8	9	6	7	8	9
99	4	4	4	4	5	5	5	5
95	5	5	5	5	6	6	6	7
90	5	5	5	5	7	7	7	7
85	6	6	6	6	8	7	8	8
80	6	6	6	7	8	8	8	9
75	6	7	7	7	8	8	9	10
70	7	7	7	8	9	9	10	10
65	7	7	7	8	9	9	10	11
60	7	7	8	9	10	10	11	11
55	7	8	8	10	10	10	11	12
50	8	8	9	10	10	11	12	13
45	8	9	10	11	11	12	13	14
40	9	9	10	11	11	12	13	14
35	9	10	11	12	12	13	14	15
30	10	11	11	13	13	13	15	16
25	10	11	12	14	13	15	16	17
20	11	12	14	15	14	15	18	18
15	12	14	15	17	16	17	19	20
10	13	16	19	20	17	18	21	22
5	17	19	21	24	20	21	24	27

This table is reprinted with permission from the JOPERD (Journal of Physical Education, Recreation & Dance), Nov-Dec, 1987, p. 67. JOPERD is a publication of the American Alliance for Health, Physical Education, Recreation and Dance, 1900 Association Drive, Reston, VA 22091-1599.

Table A.19   NCYFS II Norms by Age for the Sum of Triceps and Medial Calf Skinfolds (in Millimeters)

	Age							
	Boys				Girls			
Percentile	6	7	8	9	6	7	8	9
99	9	9	9	9	11	11	11	12
95	11	11	11	11	13	13	14	14
90	12	12	12	12	15	15	15	16
85	12	13	13	13	16	16	16	18
80	13	13	13	14	17	17	18	19
75	14	14	14	15	18	18	19	20
70	14	14	15	16	18	18	20	21
65	15	15	15	18	19	19	21	22
60	15	16	17	18	20	20	22	23
55	16	16	17	19	21	21	23	25
50	16	17	18	21	21	22	24	26
45	17	18	19	22	22	23	26	27
40	17	19	20	23	23	24	27	29
35	18	20	21	25	24	25	29	30
30	20	21	23	27	25	26	31	32
25	20	22	24	29	27	28	33	35
20	22	24	27	31	28	31	35	37
15	23	27	31	35	30	33	38	41
10	27	32	37	40	33	37	43	45
5	33	39	44	47	38	43	49	52

This table is reprinted with permission from the JOPERD (Journal of Physical Education, Recreation & Dance), Nov-Dec, 1987, p. 68. JOPERD is a publication of the American Alliance for Health, Physical Education, Recreation and Dance, 1900 Association Drive, Reston, VA 22091-1599.

Table A.20   NCYFS II Norms by Age for the Modified Pull-Ups (Number Completed)

	Age							
	Boys				Girls			
Percentile	6	7	8	9	6	7	8	9
99	25	27	38	35	24	27	25	30
95	18	20	21	25	17	20	20	20
90	15	19	20	20	13	16	17	17
85	12	15	17	20	11	14	14	15
80	11	13	15	17	10	12	12	13
75	10	13	14	15	9	11	11	12
70	9	12	13	14	9	10	11	11
65	8	11	12	13	7	9	10	10
60	7	10	11	12	7	8	9	10
55	7	9	10	11	6	8	9	9
50	6	8	10	10	6	7	8	9
45	6	8	9	10	5	7	7	8
40	5	7	8	9	5	6	6	7
35	5	6	8	8	4	5	6	6
30	4	5	7	7	4	4	5	5
25	3	4	6	6	3	4	4	4
20	3	4	5	5	2	3	4	4
15	2	3	4	4	1	2	3	2
10	1	1	3	3	0	1	1	1
5	0	0	1	2	0	0	0	0

This table is reprinted with permission from the JOPERD (Journal of Physical Education, Recreation & Dance), Nov-Dec, 1987, p. 69. JOPERD is a publication of the American Alliance for Health, Physical Education, Recreation and Dance, 1900 Association Drive, Reston, VA 22091-1599.

Physical Best Health Fitness Standards

Table A.21   Health Fitness Standards for Boys

Age	Test item					
	One-mile walk/run (min)	Sum of skinfolds (mm)	Body mass index	Sit-and-reach (cm)	Sit-ups	Pull-ups
5	13:00	12-25	13-20	25	20	1
6	12:00	12-25	13-20	25	20	1
7	11:00	12-25	13-20	25	24	1
8	10:00	12-25	14-20	25	26	1
9	10:00	12-25	14-20	25	30	1
10	9:30	12-25	14-20	25	34	1
11	9:00	12-25	15-21	25	36	2
12	9:00	12-25	15-22	25	38	2
13	8:00	12-25	16-23	25	40	3
14	7:45	12-25	16-24	25	40	4
15	7:30	12-25	17-24	25	42	5
16	7:30	12-25	18-24	25	44	5
17	7:30	12-25	18-25	25	44	5
18	7:30	12-25	18-26	25	44	5

Note: From *Physical Best* (p. 29) by American Alliance for Health, Physical Education, Recreation and Dance, 1989, Reston, VA: Author. Copyright 1989 by American Alliance for Health, Physical Education, Recreation and Dance. Reprinted with permission from American Alliance for Health, Physical Education, Recreation and Dance.

Table A.22   Health Fitness Standards for Girls

Age	One-mile walk/run (min)	Sum of skinfolds (mm)	Body mass index	Sit-and-reach (cm)	Sit-ups	Pull-ups
			Test item			
5	14:00	16-36	14-20	25	20	1
6	13:00	16-36	14-20	25	20	1
7	12:00	16-36	14-20	25	24	1
8	11:30	16-36	14-20	25	26	1
9	11:00	16-36	14-20	25	28	1
10	11:00	16-36	14-21	25	30	1
11	11:00	16-36	14-21	25	33	1
12	11:00	16-36	15-22	25	33	1
13	10:30	16-36	15-23	25	33	1
14	10:30	16-36	17-24	25	35	1
15	10:30	16-36	17-24	25	35	1
16	10:30	16-36	17-24	25	35	1
17	10:30	16-36	17-25	25	35	1
18	10:30	16-36	18-26	25	35	1

Note: From *Physical Best* (p. 28) by American Alliance for Health, Physical Education, Recreation and Dance, 1989, Reston, VA: Author. Copyright 1989 by American Alliance for Health, Physical Education, Recreation and Dance. Reprinted with permission from American Alliance for Health, Physical Education, Recreation and Dance.

The Prudential FITNESSGRAM

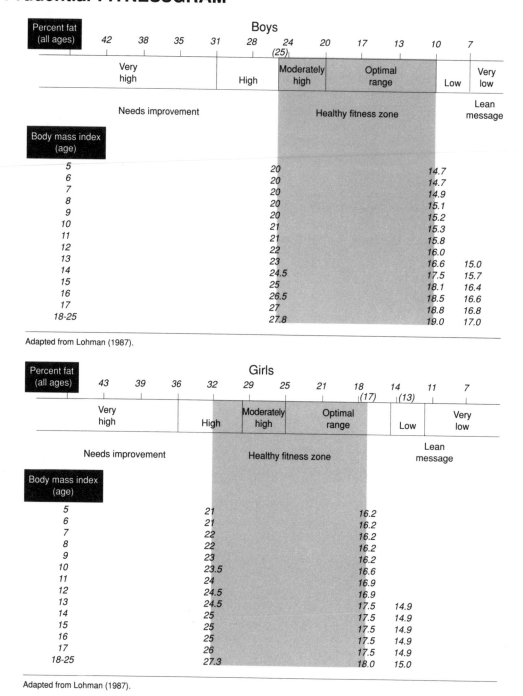

Adapted from Lohman (1987).

Adapted from Lohman (1987).

Table A.23   Standards for Healthy Fitness Zone—Boys*

Age	One mile (min:sec)		PACER (# laps)	$\dot{V}O_2max$ (ml/kg/min)		Percent fat		Body mass index	Curl-ups (# completed)	
5	Completion of		Participate in			25	10	20	2	10
6	distance. Time		run. Lap count			25	10	20	2	10
7	standards not		standards not			25	10	20	4	14
8	recommended.		recommended.			25	10	20	6	20
9						25	10	20	9	24
10	11:30	9:00	17	55	42	52	25	10	21	12	24
11	11:00	8:30	23	61	42	52	25	10	21	15	28
12	10:30	8:00	29	68	42	52	25	10	22	18	36
13	10:00	7:30	35	74	42	52	25	10	23	21	40
14	9:30	7:00	41	80	42	52	25	10	24.5	24	45
15	9:00	7:00	46	85	42	52	25	10	25	24	47
16	8:30	7:00	52	90	42	52	25	10	26.5	24	47
17	8:30	7:00	57	94	42	52	25	10	27	24	47
17+	8:30	7:00	57	94	42	52	25	10	27.8	24	47

Note on BMI column: 14.7, 14.7, 14.9, 15.1, 15.2, 15.3, 15.8, 16.0, 16.6, 17.5, 18.1, 18.5, 18.8, 19.0

(continued)

Table A.23　(*continued*)

Age	Trunk lift (in.)		Push-ups (# completed)		Modified pull-ups (# completed)		Pull-ups (# completed)		Flexed arm hang (sec)		Back saver sit-and-reach** (in.)	Shoulder stretch***
5	6	12	3	8	2	7	1	2	2	8	8	
6	6	12	3	8	2	7	1	2	2	8	8	
7	6	12	4	10	3	9	1	2	3	8	8	
8	6	12	5	13	4	11	1	2	3	10	8	
9	6	12	6	15	5	11	1	2	4	10	8	
10	9	12	7	20	5	15	1	2	4	10	8	
11	9	12	8	20	6	17	1	3	6	13	8	
12	9	12	10	20	7	20	1	3	10	15	8	
13	9	12	12	25	8	22	1	4	12	17	8	
14	9	12	14	30	9	25	2	5	15	20	8	
15	9	12	16	35	10	27	3	7	15	20	8	
16	9	12	18	35	12	30	5	8	15	20	8	
17	9	12	18	35	14	30	5	8	15	20	8	
17+	9	12	18	35	14	30	5	8	15	20	8	

*Number on left is lower end of Healthy Fitness Zone; number on right is upper end of Healthy Fitness Zone.

**Test scored Pass/Fail; must reach this distance to pass.

***Passing = Touching the fingertips together behind the back.

Note. From the Prudential FITNESSGRAM (1992). Copyright 1992 by Cooper Institute^MM. Reprinted with permission from Cooper Institute for Aerobics Research, Dallas, TX.

Table A.24   Standards for Healthy Fitness Zone—Girls*

Age	One mile (min:sec)	PACER (# laps)	V̇O₂max (ml/kg/min)	Percent fat		Body mass index	Curl-ups (# completed)	
5	Completion of	Participate in		32	17	16.2	2	10
6	distance. Time	run. Lap count		32	17	16.2	2	10
7	standards not	standards not		32	17	16.2	4	14
8	recommended.	recommended.		32	17	16.2	6	20
9				32	17	16.2	9	22
10	12:30	7	39	47	32	17	16.6	12	26
11	9:30	9	38	46	32	17	16.9	15	29
12	12:00	13	37	45	32	17	16.9	18	32
13	12:00	15	36	44	32	17	17.5	18	32
14	11:30	18	35	43	32	17	17.5	18	32
15	11:00	23	35	43	32	17	17.5	18	35
16	10:30	28	35	43	32	17	17.5	18	35
17	10:00	34	35	43	32	17	17.5	18	35
17+	10:00	34	35	43	32	17	18.0	18	35

(continued)

Table A.24 (continued)

Age	Trunk lift (in.)		Push-ups (# completed)		Modified pull-ups (# completed)		Pull-ups (# completed)		Flexed arm hang (sec)		Back saver sit-and-reach** (in.)	Shoulder stretch***
5	6	12	3	8	2	7	1	2	2	8	9	
6	6	12	3	8	2	7	1	2	2	8	9	
7	6	12	4	10	3	9	1	2	3	8	9	
8	6	12	5	13	4	11	1	2	3	10	9	
9	6	12	6	15	4	11	1	2	4	10	9	
10	9	12	7	15	4	13	1	2	4	10	9	
11	9	12	7	15	4	13	1	2	6	12	10	
12	9	12	7	15	4	13	1	2	7	12	10	
13	9	12	7	15	4	13	1	2	8	12	10	
14	9	12	7	15	4	13	1	2	8	12	10	
15	9	12	7	15	4	13	1	2	8	12	12	
16	9	12	7	15	4	13	1	2	8	12	12	
17	9	12	7	15	4	13	1	2	8	12	12	
17+	9	12	7	15	4	13	1	2	8	12	12	

*Number on left is lower end of Healthy Fitness Zone; number on right is upper end of Healthy Fitness Zone.
**Test scored Pass/Fail; must reach this distance to pass.
***Passing = Touching the fingertips together behind the back.
Note. From the Prudential FITNESSGRAM (1992). Copyright 1992 by Cooper Institute^{MM}. Reprinted with permission from Cooper Institute for Aerobics Research, Dallas, TX.

About the Authors

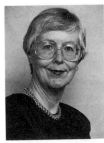

Jo Safrit is professor and chair of the Department of Health and Fitness at The American University in Washington, DC. A specialist in measurement and evaluation, she has been active in youth fitness testing in the schools for many years. She was part of the task force that developed the first health-related physical fitness test in the 1970s. She is currently a member of the Prudential FITNESSGRAM Advisory Board and the Fitness Advisory Committee of the American Alliance for Health, Physical Education, Recreation and Dance (AAHPERD).

Safrit has published papers and research on physical fitness testing. She has received many awards, including the Honor Award from the Physical Fitness Council and the Measurement and Evaluation Council and the 1994 Luther Halsey Gulick Award, the highest award bestowed by AAHPERD.

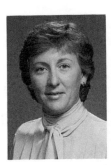

Cynthia L. Pemberton, author of chapters 6 and 7, is an associate professor in the Department of Physical Education with the University of Missouri at Kansas City. She is the 1993-94 president of the American Association for Active Lifestyles and Fitness (AAALF), an association of AAHPERD.

Focusing her research efforts on understanding motivation and physical activity in children and adults, Pemberton has published or presented more than 65 works in this area. Pemberton serves on the editorial board of the journal *Pediatric Exercise Science* and as a guest reviewer for several journals in the area of sport psychology.

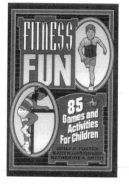
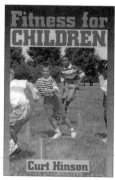
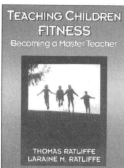
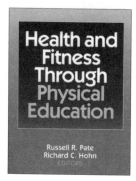
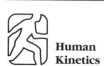